How to Read a Paper

The Basics of Evidence-Bas[...]

FIFTH EDITION

DATE DUE			

How to Read a Paper

The Basics of Evidence-Based Medicine

FIFTH EDITION

Trisha Greenhalgh
Professor of Primary Health Care
Barts and the London School of Medicine and Dentistry
Blizard Institute
London, UK

WILEY   BMJ|Books

This edition first published 2014, © 2010, 2014 by John Wiley & Sons Ltd

BMJ Books is an imprint of BMJ Publishing Group Limited, used under licence by John Wiley & Sons.

Registered office: John Wiley & Sons, Ltd, The Atrium, Southern Gate, Chichester, West Sussex,
PO19 8SQ, UK

Editorial offices: 9600 Garsington Road, Oxford, OX4 2DQ, UK
The Atrium, Southern Gate, Chichester, West Sussex, PO19 8SQ, UK
111 River Street, Hoboken, NJ 07030-5774, USA

For details of our global editorial offices, for customer services and for information about how to apply
for permission to reuse the copyright material in this book please see our website at
www.wiley.com/wiley-blackwell

The right of the author to be identified as the author of this work has been asserted in accordance with
the UK Copyright, Designs and Patents Act 1988.

Library of Congress Cataloging-in-Publication Data

Greenhalgh, Trisha, author.
  How to read a paper : the basics of evidence-based medicine / Trisha Greenhalgh. – Fifth edition.
     p. ; cm.
  Includes bibliographical references and index.
  ISBN 978-1-118-80096-6 (pbk.)
  I. Title.
  [DNLM: 1. Evidence-Based Practice. 2. Journalism, Medical. 3. Research. WB 102.5]
  R118.6
  610.72 – dc23

                                                                                    2013038474

A catalogue record for this book is available from the British Library.

Wiley also publishes its books in a variety of electronic formats. Some content that appears in print may
not be available in electronic books.

Cover design by Meaden Creative

Typeset in 9.5/12 pt MinionPro by Laserwords Private Limited, Chennai, India
Printed and bound in Malaysia by Vivar Printing Sdn Bhd

2   2014

In November 1995, my friend Ruth Holland,
book reviews editor of the *British Medical Journal*,
suggested that I write a book to demystify the important
but often inaccessible subject of evidence-based medicine.
She provided invaluable comments on earlier drafts of the
manuscript, but was tragically killed in a train crash on
August 8, 1996. This book is dedicated to her memory.

Contents

Foreword to the first edition by Professor Sir David Weatherall

Not surprisingly, the wide publicity given to what is now called *evidence-based medicine* has been greeted with mixed reactions by those who are involved in the provision of patient care. The bulk of the medical profession appears to be slightly hurt by the concept, suggesting as it does that until recently all medical practice was what Lewis Thomas has described as a frivolous and irresponsible kind of human experimentation, based on nothing but trial and error, and usually resulting in precisely that sequence. On the other hand, politicians and those who administrate our health services have greeted the notion with enormous glee. They had suspected all along that doctors were totally uncritical and now they had it on paper. Evidence-based medicine came as a gift from the gods because, at least as they perceived it, its implied efficiency must inevitably result in cost saving.

The concept of controlled clinical trials and evidence-based medicine is not new, however. It is recorded that Frederick II, Emperor of the Romans and King of Sicily and Jerusalem, who lived from 1192 to 1250 AD, and who was interested in the effects of exercise on digestion, took two knights and gave them identical meals. One was then sent out hunting and the other ordered to bed. At the end of several hours, he killed both and examined the contents of their alimentary canals; digestion had proceeded further in the stomach of the sleeping knight. In the 17th century, Jan Baptista van Helmont, a physician and philosopher, became sceptical of the practice of blood-letting. Hence he proposed what was almost certainly the first clinical trial involving large numbers, randomisation and statistical analysis. This involved taking 200–500 poor people, dividing them into two groups by casting lots, and protecting one from phlebotomy while allowing the other to be treated with as much blood-letting as his colleagues thought appropriate. The number of funerals in each group would be used to assess the efficacy of blood-letting. History does not record why this splendid experiment was never carried out.

If modern scientific medicine can be said to have had a beginning it was in Paris in the mid-19th century and where it had its roots in the work and teachings of Pierre Charles Alexandre Louis. Louis introduced statistical analysis to the evaluation of medical treatment and, incidentally, showed that blood-letting was a valueless form of treatment, although this did not change the habits of the physicians of the time, or for many years to come. Despite this pioneering work, few clinicians on either side of the Atlantic urged that trials of clinical outcome should be adopted, although the principles of numerically based experimental design were enunciated in the 1920s by the geneticist Ronald Fisher. The field only started to make a major impact on clinical practice after the Second World War following the seminal work of Sir Austin Bradford Hill and the British epidemiologists who followed him, notably Richard Doll and Archie Cochrane.

But although the idea of evidence-based medicine is not new, modern disciples like David Sackett and his colleagues are doing a great service to clinical practice, not just by popularising the idea but by bringing home to clinicians the notion that it is not a dry academic subject but more a way of thinking that should permeate every aspect of medical practice. While much of it is based on mega-trials and meta-analyses, it should also be used to influence almost everything that a doctor does. After all, the medical profession has been brain-washed for years by examiners in medical schools and Royal Colleges to believe that there is only one way of examining a patient. Our bedside rituals could do with as much critical evaluation as our operations and drug regimes; the same goes for almost every aspect of doctoring.

As clinical practice becomes busier, and time for reading and reflection becomes even more precious, the ability effectively to peruse the medical literature and, in the future, to become familiar with a knowledge of best practice from modern communication systems, will be essential skills for doctors. In this lively book, Trisha Greenhalgh provides an excellent approach to how to make best use of medical literature and the benefits of evidence-based medicine. It should have equal appeal for first year medical students and grey-haired consultants, and deserves to be read widely.

With increasing years, the privilege of being invited to write a foreword to a book by one's ex-students becomes less of a rarity. Trisha Greenhalgh was the kind of medical student who never let her teachers get away with a loose thought and this inquiring attitude seems to have flowered over the years; this is a splendid and timely book and I wish it all the success it deserves. After all, the concept of evidence-based medicine is nothing more than the state of mind that every clinical teacher hopes to develop in their students; Dr Green-halgh's sceptical but constructive approach to medical literature suggests that such a happy outcome is possible at least once in the lifetime of a professor of medicine.

DJ Weatherall
Oxford

Preface to the first edition: do you need to read this book?

This book is intended for anyone, whether medically qualified or not, who wishes to find their way into the medical literature, assess the scientific validity and practical relevance of the articles they find, and, where appropriate, put the results into practice. These skills constitute the basics of evidence-based medicine.

I hope this book will help you to read and interpret medical papers better. I hope, in addition, to convey a further message, which is this. Many of the descriptions given by cynics of what evidence-based medicine is (the glorification of things that can be measured without regard for the usefulness or accuracy of what is measured, the uncritical acceptance of published numerical data, the preparation of all-encompassing guidelines by self-appointed 'experts' who are out of touch with real medicine, the debasement of clinical freedom through the imposition of rigid and dogmatic clinical protocols, and the over-reliance on simplistic, inappropriate and often incorrect economic analyses) are actually criticisms of what the evidence-based medicine movement is fighting *against*, rather than of what it represents.

Do not, however, think of me as an evangelist for the gospel according to evidence-based medicine. I believe that the science of finding, evaluating and implementing the results of medical research can, and often does, make patient care more objective, more logical, and more cost-effective. If I didn't believe that, I wouldn't spend so much of my time teaching it and trying, as a general practitioner, to practise it. Nevertheless, I believe that when applied in a vacuum (that is, in the absence of common sense and without regard to the individual circumstances and priorities of the person being offered treatment or to the complex nature of clinical practice and policymaking), 'evidence-based' decision-making is a reductionist process with a real potential for harm.

Finally, you should note that I am neither an epidemiologist nor a statistician, but a person who reads papers and who has developed a pragmatic (and at times unconventional) system for testing their merits. If you wish to pursue the epidemiological or statistical themes covered in this book, I would encourage you to move on to a more definitive text, references for which you will find at the end of each chapter.

Trisha Greenhalgh

Preface to the fifth edition

When I wrote this book in 1996, evidence-based medicine was a bit of an unknown quantity. A handful of academics (including me) were already enthusiastic and had begun running 'training the trainers' courses to disseminate what we saw as a highly logical and systematic approach to clinical practice. Others – certainly the majority of clinicians – were convinced that this was a passing fad that was of limited importance and would never catch on. I wrote *How to Read a Paper* for two reasons. First, students on my own courses were asking for a simple introduction to the principles presented in what was then known as *Dave Sackett's Big Red Book* (Sackett DL, Haynes RB, Guyatt GH, Tugwell P. *Clinical epidemiology – a basic science for clinical medicine*. London: Little, Brown & Co., 1991) – an outstanding and inspirational volume that was already in its fourth reprint, but which some novices apparently found a hard read. Second, it was clear to me that many of the critics of evidence-based medicine didn't really understand what they were dismissing – and that until they did, serious debate on the political, ideological and pedagogical place of evidence-based medicine as a discipline could not begin.

I am of course delighted that *How to Read a Paper* has become a standard reader in many medical and nursing schools, and that it has so far been translated into French, German, Italian, Spanish, Portuguese, Chinese, Polish, Japanese, Czech and Russian. I am also delighted that what was so recently a fringe subject in academia has been well and truly mainstreamed in clinical service. In the UK, for example, it is now a contractual requirement for all doctors, nurses and pharmacists to practise (and for managers to manage) according to best research evidence.

In the 18 years since the first edition of this book was published, evidence-based medicine has waxed and waned in popularity. Hundreds of textbooks and tens of thousands of journal articles now offer different angles on the 'basics of EBM' covered briefly in the chapters that follow. An increasing number of these sources point out genuine limitations of evidence-based medicine in certain contexts. Others look at evidence-based medicine as a social movement – a 'bandwagon' that took off at a particular time (the 1990s) and place (North America) and spread dramatically quickly with all sorts of knock-on effects for particular interest groups.

When preparing this fifth edition, I was once again minded not to change too much apart from updating the examples and the reference lists, as there is clearly still room on the bookshelves for a no-frills introductory text. In the last (fourth edition), I also added two new chapters (on quality improvement and complex interventions), and in this latest edition I have added two more – one on applying evidence-based medicine with patients (the science of shared decision making) and another on common criticisms of EBM and responses to those. As ever, I would welcome any feedback that will help make the text more accurate, readable and practical.

Trisha Greenhalgh
January 2014

Acknowledgements

I am not by any standards an expert on all of the subjects covered in this book (in particular, I am very bad at sums), and I am grateful to the people listed here for help along the way. I am, however, the final author of every chapter, and responsibility for any inaccuracies is mine alone.

1. To Professor Sir Andy Haines and Professor Dave Sackett who introduced me to the subject of evidence-based medicine and encouraged me to write about it.

2. To the late Dr Anna Donald, who broadened my outlook through valuable discussions on the implications and uncertainties of this evolving discipline.

3. To Jeanette Buckingham of the University of Alberta, Canada, for invaluable input to Chapter 2.

4. To various expert advisers and proofreaders who had direct input to this new edition or who advised me on previous editions.

5. To the many readers, too numerous to mention individually, who took time to write in and point out both typographical and factual errors in previous editions. As a result of their contributions, I have learnt a great deal (especially about statistics) and the book has been improved in many ways. Some of the earliest critics of *How to Read a Paper* have subsequently worked with me on my teaching courses in evidence-based practice; several have co-authored other papers or book chapters with me, and one or two have become personal friends.

6. To the authors and publishers of articles who gave permission for me to reproduce figures or tables. Details are given in the text.

7. To my followers on Twitter who proposed numerous ideas, constructive criticisms and responses to my suggestions when I was preparing the fifth edition of this book. By the way, you should try Twitter as a source of evidence-based information. Follow me on @trishgreenhalgh – and while you're at it you could try the Cochrane Collaboration on @cochrancollab, Ben Goldacre on @bengoldacre, Carl Heneghan from the Oxford Centre

for Evidence Based Medicine on @cebmblog and the UK National Institute for Health and Care Excellence on @nicecomms.

Thanks also to my husband, Dr Fraser Macfarlane, for his unfailing support for my academic work and writing. My sons Rob and Al had not long been born when the first edition of this book was being written. It is a source of great pride to me that they have now read the book, applied its messages in their own developing scientific careers (one in medicine) and made suggestions on how to improve it.

Chapter 1 Why read papers at all?

Does 'evidence-based medicine' simply mean 'reading papers in medical journals'?

Evidence-based medicine (EBM) is much more than just reading papers. According to the most widely quoted definition, it is 'the conscientious, explicit and judicious use of current best evidence in making decisions about the care of individual patients' [1]. I find this definition very useful but it misses out what for me is a very important aspect of the subject – and that is the use of mathematics. Even if you know almost nothing about EBM, you probably know it talks a lot about numbers and ratios! Anna Donald and I decided to be upfront about this in our own teaching, and proposed this alternative definition:

> Evidence-based medicine is the use of mathematical estimates of the risk of benefit and harm, derived from high-quality research on population samples, to inform clinical decision-making in the diagnosis, investigation or management of individual patients.

The defining feature of EBM, then, is the use of figures derived from research on *populations* to inform decisions about *individuals*. This, of course, begs the question 'What is research?' – for which a reasonably accurate answer might be 'Focused, systematic enquiry aimed at generating new knowledge'. In later chapters, I will explain how this definition can help you distinguish genuine research (which should inform your practice) from the poor-quality endeavours of well-meaning amateurs (which you should politely ignore).

If you follow an evidence-based approach to clinical decision-making, therefore, all sorts of issues relating to your patients (or, if you work in public

How to Read a Paper: The Basics of Evidence-Based Medicine, Fifth Edition. Trisha Greenhalgh.
© 2014 John Wiley & Sons, Ltd. Published 2014 by John Wiley & Sons, Ltd.

health medicine, issues relating to groups of people) will prompt you to ask questions about scientific evidence, seek answers to those questions in a systematic way and alter your practice accordingly.

You might ask questions, for example, about a patient's symptoms ('In a 34-year-old man with left-sided chest pain, what is the probability that there is a serious heart problem, and, if there is, will it show up on a resting ECG?'), about physical or diagnostic signs ('In an otherwise uncomplicated child-birth, does the presence of meconium [indicating fetal bowel movement] in the amniotic fluid indicate significant deterioration in the physiological state of the fetus?'), about the prognosis of an illness ('If a previously well two-year-old has a short fit associated with a high temperature, what is the chance that she will subsequently develop epilepsy?'), about therapy ('In patients with an acute coronary syndrome [heart attack], are the risks associated with thrombolytic drugs [clot busters] outweighed by the benefits, whatever the patient's age, sex and ethnic origin?'), about cost-effectiveness ('Is the cost of this new anti-cancer drug justified, compared with other ways of spending limited healthcare resources?'), about patients' preferences ('In an 87-year-old woman with intermittent atrial fibrillation and a recent transient ischaemic attack, does the inconvenience of warfarin therapy outweigh the risks of not taking it?'), and about a host of other aspects of health and health services.

Professor Sackett, in the opening editorial of the very first issue of the journal *Evidence-Based Medicine* summarised the essential steps in the emerging science of EBM [2]:

1. To convert our information needs into answerable questions (i.e. to formulate the problem);
2. To track down, with maximum efficiency, the best evidence with which to answer these questions – which may come from the clinical examination, the diagnostic laboratory, the published literature or other sources;
3. To appraise the evidence critically (i.e. weigh it up) to assess its validity (closeness to the truth) and usefulness (clinical applicability);
4. To implement the results of this appraisal in our clinical practice;
5. To evaluate our performance.

Hence, EBM requires you not only to read papers but to read the *right* papers at the right time, and then to alter your behaviour (and, what is often more difficult, influence the behaviour of other people) in the light of what you have found. I am concerned that how-to-do-it courses in EBM too often concentrate on the third of these five steps (critical appraisal) to the exclusion of all the others. Yet if you have asked the wrong question or sought answers from the wrong sources, you might as well not read any papers at all. Equally, all your training in search techniques and critical appraisal will go to waste if you do not put at least as much effort into implementing valid evidence and measuring progress towards your goals as you do into reading the paper. A few years ago, I added three more stages to Sackett's five-stage model to incorporate the patient's perspective: the resulting eight stages, which I have called a *context-sensitive checklist for evidence-based practice*, are shown in Appendix 1 [3].

If I were to be pedantic about the title of this book, these broader aspects of EBM should not even get a mention here. But I hope you would have demanded your money back if I had omitted the final section of this chapter (Before you start: formulate the problem), Chapter 2 (Searching the literature), Chapter 15 (Implementing evidence-based practice) and Chapter 16 (Applying evidence with patients). Chapters 3–14 describe step three of the EBM process: critical appraisal – that is, what you should do when you actually have the paper in front of you. Chapter 16 deals with common criticisms of EBM.

Incidentally, if you are computer literate and want to explore the subject of EBM on the Internet, you could try the websites listed in Box 1.1. If you're not, don't worry at this stage, but do put learning/use web-based resources to on your to-do list. Don't worry either when you discover that there are over 1000 websites dedicated to EBM – they all offer very similar material and you certainly don't need to visit them all.

Box 1.1 Web-based resources for Evidence-based medicine

Oxford Centre for Evidence-Based Medicine: A well-kept website from Oxford, UK, containing a wealth of resources and links for EBM. http://cebm.net.

National Institute for Health and Care Excellence: This UK-based website, which is also popular outside the UK, links to evidence-based guidelines and topic reviews. http://www.nice.org.uk/.

National Health Service (NHS) Centre for Reviews and Dissemination: The site for downloading the high-quality evidence-based reviews is part of the UK National Institute for Health Research – a good starting point for looking for evidence on complex questions such as 'what should we do about obesity?' http://www.york.ac.uk/inst/crd/.

Clinical Evidence: An online handbook of best evidence for clinical decisions such as 'what's the best current treatment for atrial fibrillation?' Produced by BMJ Publishing Group. http://clinicalevidence.bmj.com.

Why do people sometimes groan when you mention evidence-based medicine?

Critics of EBM might define it as 'the tendency of a group of young, confident and highly numerate medical academics to belittle the performance of experienced clinicians using a combination of epidemiological jargon and statistical sleight-of-hand' or 'the argument, usually presented with near-evangelistic zeal, that no health-related action should ever be taken by a doctor, a nurse, a purchaser of health services, or a policymaker, unless and until the results of several large and expensive research trials have appeared in print and approved by a committee of experts'.

The resentment amongst some health professionals towards the EBM movement is mostly a reaction to the implication that doctors (and nurses, midwives, physiotherapists and other health professionals) were functionally illiterate until they were shown the light, and that the few who weren't illiterate wilfully ignored published medical evidence. Anyone who works face-to-face with patients knows how often it is necessary to seek new information before making a clinical decision. Doctors have spent time in libraries since libraries were invented. In general, we don't put a patient on a new drug without evidence that it is likely to work. Apart from anything else, such off-licence use of medication is, strictly speaking, illegal. Surely we have all been practising EBM for years, except when we were deliberately bluffing (using the 'placebo' effect for good medical reasons), or when we were ill, overstressed or consciously being lazy?

Well, no, we haven't. There have been a number of surveys on the behaviour of doctors, nurses and related professionals. It was estimated in the 1970s in the USA that only around 10–20% of all health technologies then available (i.e. drugs, procedures, operations, etc.) were evidence-based; that figure improved to 21% in 1990, according to official US statistics [4]. Studies of the interventions offered to consecutive series of patients suggested that 60–90% of clinical decisions, depending on the specialty, were 'evidence-based' [5]. But as I have argued elsewhere, such studies had methodological limitations [3]. Apart from anything else, they were undertaken in specialised units and looked at the practice of world experts in EBM; hence, the figures arrived at can hardly be generalised beyond their immediate setting (see section 'Whom is the study about?'). In all probability, we are still selling our patients short quite most of the time.

A recent large survey by an Australian team looked at 1000 patients treated for the 22 most commonly seen conditions in a primary care setting. The researchers found that whilst 90% of patients received evidence-based care for coronary heart disease, only 13% did so for alcohol dependence [6].

Furthermore, the extent to which any individual practitioner provided evidence-based care varied in the sample from 32% of the time to 86% of the time. These findings suggest room for improvement all round.

Let's take a look at the various approaches that health professionals use to reach their decisions in reality – all of which are examples of what EBM *isn't*.

Decision-making by anecdote

When I was a medical student, I occasionally joined the retinue of a distinguished professor as he made his daily ward rounds. On seeing a new patient, he would enquire about the patient's symptoms, turn to the massed ranks of juniors around the bed, and relate the story of a similar patient encountered a few years previously. 'Ah, yes. I remember we gave her such-and-such, and she was fine after that'. He was cynical, often rightly, about new drugs and technologies and his clinical acumen was second to none. Nevertheless, it had taken him 40 years to accumulate his expertise, and the largest medical textbook of all – the collection of cases that were outside his personal experience – was forever closed to him.

Anecdote (storytelling) has an important place in clinical practice [7]. Psychologists have shown that students acquire the skills of medicine, nursing and so on by memorising what was wrong with particular patients, and what happened to them, in the form of stories or 'illness scripts'. Stories about patients are the unit of analysis (i.e. the thing we study) in grand rounds and teaching sessions. Clinicians glean crucial information from patients' illness narratives – most crucially, perhaps, what being ill *means* to the patient. And experienced doctors and nurses rightly take account of the accumulated 'illness scripts' of all their previous patients when managing subsequent patients. But that doesn't mean simply doing the same for patient B as you did for patient A if your treatment worked, and doing precisely the opposite if it didn't!

The dangers of decision-making by anecdote are well illustrated by considering the risk–benefit ratio of drugs and medicines. In my first pregnancy, I developed severe vomiting and was given the anti-sickness drug prochlorperazine (Stemetil). Within minutes, I went into an uncontrollable and very distressing neurological spasm. Two days later, I had recovered fully from this idiosyncratic reaction, but I have never prescribed the drug since, even though the estimated prevalence of neurological reactions to prochlorperazine is only one in several thousand cases. Conversely, it is tempting to dismiss the possibility of rare but potentially serious adverse effects from familiar drugs – such as thrombosis on the contraceptive pill – when one has never encountered such problems in oneself or one's patients.

We clinicians would not be human if we ignored our personal clinical experiences, but we would be better to base our decisions on the collective experience of thousands of clinicians treating millions of patients, rather than on what we as individuals have seen and felt. Chapter 5 (Statistics for the non-statistician) describes some more objective methods, such as the number needed to treat (NNT), for deciding whether a particular drug (or other intervention) is likely to do a patient significant good or harm.

When the EBM movement was still in its infancy, Sackett emphasised that evidence-based practice was no threat to old-fashioned clinical experience or judgement [1]. The question of *how* clinicians can manage to be both 'evidence-based' (i.e. systematically informing their decisions by research evidence) and 'narrative-based' (i.e. embodying all the richness of their accumulated clinical anecdotes and treating each patient's problem as a unique illness story rather than as a 'case of X') is a difficult one to address philosophically, and beyond the scope of this book. The interested reader might like to look up two articles I've written on this topic [8, 9].

Decision-making by press cutting

For the first 10 years after I qualified, I kept an expanding file of papers that I had ripped out of my medical weeklies before binning the less interesting parts. If an article or editorial seemed to have something new to say, I consciously altered my clinical practice in line with its conclusions. All children with suspected urinary tract infections should be sent for scans of the kidneys to exclude congenital abnormalities, said one article, so I began referring anyone under the age of 16 with urinary symptoms for specialist investigations. The advice was in print, and it was recent, so it must surely replace what had been standard practice – in this case, referring only the small minority of such children who display 'atypical' features [10].

This approach to clinical decision-making is still very common. How many doctors do you know who justify their approach to a particular clinical problem by citing the results section of a single published study, even though they could not tell you anything at all about the methods used to obtain those results? Was the trial randomised and controlled (see section 'Cross-sectional surveys')? How many patients, of what age, sex and disease severity, were involved (see section 'Whom is the study about?')? How many withdrew from ('dropped out of') the study, and why (see section 'Were preliminary statistical questions addressed?')? By what criteria were patients judged cured (see section 'Surrogate endpoints')? If the findings of the study appeared to contradict those of other researchers, what attempt was made to validate (confirm) and replicate (repeat) them (see section 'Ten questions to ask about a paper that claims to validate a diagnostic or screening test')? Were the statistical tests that allegedly proved the authors' point appropriately chosen and correctly performed (see Chapter 5)? Has the patient's perspective been systematically sought and incorporated via a shared decision-making tool (see Chapter 16)? Doctors (and nurses, midwifes, medical managers, psychologists, medical students and consumer activists) who like to cite the results of medical research studies have a responsibility to ensure that they first go through a checklist of questions like these (more of which are listed in Appendix 1).

Decision-making by GOBSAT (good old boys sat around a table)

When I wrote the first edition of this book in the mid-1990s, the commonest sort of guideline was what was known as a *consensus statement* – the fruits of a weekend's hard work by a dozen or so eminent experts who had been shut in a luxury hotel, usually at the expense of a drug company. Such 'GOBSAT (good old boys sat around a table) guidelines' often fell out of the medical freebies (free medical journals and other 'information sheets' sponsored directly or indirectly by the pharmaceutical industry) as pocket-sized booklets replete with potted recommendations and at-a-glance management guides. But who says the advice given in a set of guidelines, a punchy editorial or an amply referenced overview is correct?

Professor Mulrow [11], one of the founders of the science of systematic review (see Chapter 9) showed a few years ago that experts in a particular clinical field are *less* likely to provide an objective review of all the available evidence than a non-expert who approaches the literature with unbiased eyes. In extreme cases, an 'expert opinion' may consist simply of the lifelong bad habits and personal press cuttings of an ageing clinician, and a gaggle of such experts would simply multiply the misguided views of any one of them. Table 1.1 gives examples of practices that were at one time widely accepted as good clinical practice (and which would have made it into the GOBSAT guideline of the day), but which have subsequently been discredited by high-quality clinical trials.

Chapter 9 takes you through a checklist for assessing whether a 'systematic review of the evidence' produced to support recommendations for practice or policymaking really merits the description, and Chapter 10 discusses the harm that can be done by applying guidelines that are not evidence-based. It is a major achievement of the EBM movement that almost no guideline these days is produced by GOBSAT!

Decision-making by cost-minimisation

The popular press tends to be horrified when they learn that a treatment has been withheld from a patient for reasons of cost. Managers, politicians and, increasingly, doctors can count on being pilloried when a child with a rare

Table 1.1 Examples of harmful practices once strongly supported by 'expert opinion'

Approximate time period	Clinical practice accepted by experts of the day	Practice shown to be harmful in	Impact on clinical practice
From 500 BC	Bloodletting (for just about any acute illness)	1820[a]	Bloodletting ceased around 1910
1957	Thalidomide for 'morning sickness' in early pregnancy, which led to the birth of over 8000 severely malformed babies worldwide	1960	The teratogenic effects of this drug were so dramatic that thalidomide was rapidly withdrawn when the first case report appeared
From at least 1900	Bed rest for acute low back pain	1986	Many doctors still advise people with back pain to 'rest up'
1960s	Benzodiazepines (e.g. diazepam) for mild anxiety and insomnia, initially marketed as 'non-addictive' but subsequently shown to cause severe dependence and withdrawal symptoms	1975	Benzodiazepine prescribing for these indications fell in the 1990s
1970s	Intravenous lignocaine in acute myocardial infarction, with a view to preventing arrhythmias, subsequently shown to have no overall benefit and in some cases to cause fatal arrhythmias	1974	Lignocaine continued to be given routinely until the mid-1980s
Late 1990s	Cox-2 inhibitors (a new class of non-steroidal anti-inflammatory drug), introduced for the treatment of arthritis, were later shown to increase the risk of heart attack and stroke	2004	Cox-2 inhibitors for pain were quickly withdrawn following some high-profile legal cases in the USA, although new uses for cancer treatment (where risks may be outweighed by benefits) are now being explored

[a] Interestingly, bloodletting was probably the first practice for which a randomised controlled trial was suggested. The physician van Helmont issued this challenge to his colleagues as early as 1662: *'Let us take 200 or 500 poor people that have fevers. Let us cast lots, that one half of them may fall to my share, and the others to yours. I will cure them without blood-letting, but you do as you know – and we shall see how many funerals both of us shall have'* [12]. I am grateful to Matthias Egger for drawing my attention to this example.

cancer is not sent to a specialist unit in America or a frail old lady is denied a drug to stop her visual loss from macular degeneration. Yet in the real world, all healthcare is provided from a limited budget and it is increasingly recognised that clinical decisions must take into account the economic costs of a given intervention. As Chapter 11 argues, clinical decision-making *purely* on the grounds of cost ('cost-minimisation' – purchasing the cheapest option with no regard to how effective it is) is generally ethically unjustified, and we are right to object vocally when this occurs.

Expensive interventions should not, however, be justified simply because they are new, or because they ought to work in theory, or because the only alternative is to do nothing – but because they are very likely to save life or significantly improve its quality. How, though, can the benefits of a hip replacement in a 75-year-old be meaningfully compared with that of cholesterol-lowering drugs in a middle-aged man or infertility investigations for a couple in their twenties? Somewhat counter-intuitively, there is no self-evident set of ethical principles or analytical tools that we can use to match limited resources to unlimited demand. As you will see in Chapter 11, the much-derided quality-adjusted life year (QALY), and similar utility-based units are simply attempts to lend some objectivity to the illogical but unavoidable comparison of apples with oranges in the field of human suffering. In the United Kingdom, the National Institute for Health and Care Excellence (see www.nice.org.uk) seeks to develop both evidence-based guidelines and fair allocation of NHS resources.

There is one more reason why some people find the term *evidence-based medicine* unpalatable. This chapter has argued that EBM is about coping with change, not about knowing all the answers before you start. In other words, it is not so much about what you have read in the past but about how you go about identifying and meeting your ongoing learning needs and applying your knowledge appropriately and consistently in new clinical situations. Doctors who were brought up in the old school style of never admitting ignorance may find it hard to accept that a major element of scientific uncertainty exists in practically every clinical encounter, although in most cases, the clinician fails to identify the uncertainty or to articulate it in terms of an answerable question (see next section). If you are interested in the research evidence on doctors' [lack of] questioning behaviour, see an excellent review by Swinglehurst [13].

The fact that none of us – not even the cleverest or most experienced – can answer all the questions that arise in the average clinical encounter means that the 'expert' is more fallible than he or she was traditionally cracked up to be. An evidence-based approach to ward rounds may turn the traditional medical hierarchy on its head when the staff nurse or junior doctor produces new evidence that challenges what the consultant taught everyone last week.

For some senior clinicians, learning the skills of critical appraisal is the least of their problems in adjusting to an evidence-based teaching style!

Having defended EBM against all the standard arguments put forward by clinicians, I should confess to being sympathetic to many of the more sophisticated arguments put forward by philosophers and social scientists. Such arguments, summarised in Chapter 17 (new for this edition), address the nature of knowledge and the question of how much medicine really rests on decisions at all. But please don't turn to that chapter (which is, philosophically speaking, a 'hard read') until you have fully grasped the basic arguments in the first few chapters of this book – or you risk becoming confused!

Before you start: formulate the problem

When I ask my medical students to write me an essay about high blood pressure, they often produce long, scholarly and essentially correct statements on what high blood pressure is, what causes it and what the different treatment options are. On the day they hand their essays in, most of them know far more about high blood pressure than I do. They are certainly aware that high blood pressure is the single most common cause of stroke, and that detecting and treating everyone's high blood pressure would cut the incidence of stroke by almost half. Most of them are aware that stroke, although devastating when it happens, is a fairly rare event, and that blood pressure tablets have side effects such as tiredness, dizziness, impotence and getting 'caught short' when a long way from the lavatory.

But when I ask my students a practical question such as 'Mrs Jones has developed light-headedness on these blood pressure tablets and she wants to stop all medication; what would you advise her to do?', they are often foxed. They sympathise with Mrs Jones' predicament, but they cannot distil from their pages of close-written text the one thing that Mrs Jones needs to know. As Smith (paraphrasing TS Eliot) asked a few years ago in a BMJ editorial: 'Where is the wisdom we have lost in knowledge, and the knowledge we have lost in information?'[14].

Experienced clinicians might think they can answer Mrs Jones' question from their own personal experience. As I argued in the previous section, few of them would be right. And even if they were right on this occasion, they would still need an overall system for converting the rag-bag of information about a patient (an ill-defined set of symptoms, physical signs, test results and knowledge of what happened to this patient or a similar patient last time), the particular values and preferences (utilities) of the patient and other things that could be relevant (a hunch, a half-remembered article, the opinion of a more experienced colleague or a paragraph discovered by chance while flicking through a textbook) into a succinct summary of what the problem is and what specific additional items of information we need to solve that problem.

Sackett and colleagues, in a book subsequently revised by Straus [15], have helped us by dissecting the parts of a good clinical question:

- First, define precisely *whom* the question is about (i.e. ask 'How would I describe a group of patients similar to this one?').
- Next, define *which* manoeuvre you are considering in this patient or population (e.g. a drug treatment), and, if necessary, a comparison manoeuvre (e.g. placebo or current standard therapy).
- Finally, define the desired (or undesired) *outcome* (e.g. reduced mortality, better quality of life, and overall cost savings to the health service).

The second step may not concern a drug treatment, surgical operation or other intervention. The manoeuvre could, for example, be the exposure to a putative carcinogen (something that might cause cancer) or the detection of a particular surrogate endpoint in a blood test or other investigation. (A surrogate endpoint, as section 'Surrogate endpoints' explains, is something that predicts, or is said to predict, the later development or progression of disease. In reality, there are very few tests that reliably act as crystal balls for patients' medical future. The statement 'The doctor looked at the test results and told me I had six months to live' usually reflects either poor memory or irresponsible doctoring!) In both these cases, the 'outcome' would be the development of cancer (or some other disease) several years later. In most clinical problems with individual patients, however, the 'manoeuvre' consists of a specific intervention initiated by a health professional.

Thus, in Mrs Jones's case, we might ask, 'In a 68-year-old white woman with essential (i.e. common or garden) hypertension (high blood pressure), no coexisting illness, and no significant past medical history, whose blood pressure is currently X/Y, do the benefits of continuing therapy with bendroflumethiazide (chiefly, reduced risk of stroke) outweigh the inconvenience?'. Note that in framing the specific question, we have already established that Mrs Jones has never had a heart attack, stroke or early warning signs such as transient paralysis or loss of vision. If she had, her risk of subsequent stroke would be much higher and we would, rightly, load the risk–benefit equation to reflect this.

In order to answer the question we have posed, we must determine not just the risk of stroke in untreated hypertension but also the likely reduction in that risk which we can expect with drug treatment. This is, in fact, a rephrasing of a more general question (do the benefits of treatment in this case outweigh the risks?) which we should have asked before we prescribed bendroflumethiazide to Mrs Jones in the first place, and which all doctors should, of course, ask themselves every time they reach for their prescription pad.

Remember that Mrs Jones' alternative to staying on this particular drug is not necessarily to take no drugs at all; there may be other drugs with equivalent efficacy but less disabling side effects (as Chapter 6 argues, too many clinical trials of new drugs compare the product with placebo rather than with the best available alternative), or non-medical treatments such as exercise, salt restriction, homeopathy or yoga. Not all of these approaches would help Mrs Jones or be acceptable to her, but it would be quite appropriate to seek evidence as to *whether* they might help her – especially if she was asking to try one or more of these remedies.

We will probably find answers to some of these questions in the medical literature, and Chapter 2 describes how to search for relevant papers once you have formulated the problem. But before you start, give one last thought to your patient with high blood pressure. In order to determine her personal priorities (how does she value a 10% reduction in her risk of stroke in 5 years' time compared to the inability to go shopping unaccompanied today?), you will need to approach Mrs Jones, not a blood pressure specialist or the Medline database! Chapter 16 sets out some structured approaches for doing this.

Exercise 1

1. Go back to the fourth paragraph in this chapter, where examples of clinical questions are given. Decide whether each of these is a properly focused question in terms of
   (a) the patient or problem;
   (b) the manoeuvre (intervention, prognostic marker, exposure);
   (c) the comparison manoeuvre, if appropriate;
   (d) the clinical outcome.
2. Now try the following:
   (a) A 5-year-old child has been on high-dose topical steroids for severe eczema since the age of 20 months. The mother believes that the steroids are stunting the child's growth, and wishes to change to homeopathic treatment. What information does the dermatologist need to decide (i) whether she is right about the topical steroids and (ii) whether homeopathic treatment will help this child?
   (b) A woman who is 9 weeks pregnant calls out her general practitioner (GP) because of abdominal pain and bleeding. A previous ultrasound

scan showed that the pregnancy was not ectopic. The GP decides that she might be having a miscarriage and tells her she must go into hospital for a scan and, possibly, an operation to clear out the womb. The woman is reluctant. What information do they both need in order to establish whether hospital admission is medically necessary?

(c) A 48-year-old man presents to a private physician complaining of low back pain. The physician administers an injection of corticosteroid. Sadly, the man develops fungal meningitis and dies. What information is needed to determine both the benefits and the potential harms of steroid injections in low back pain, in order to advise patients on the risk-benefit balance?

References

1 Sackett DL, Rosenberg WM, Gray J, et al. Evidence based medicine: what it is and what it isn't. BMJ: British Medical Journal 1996;**312**(7023):71.

2 Sackett DL, Haynes RB. On the need for evidence-based medicine. Evidence Based Medicine 1995;**1**(1):4–5.

3 Greenhalgh T. Is my practice evidence-based? BMJ: British Medical Journal 1996;**313**(7063):957.

4 Dubinsky M, Ferguson JH. Analysis of the National Institutes of Health Medicare coverage assessment. International Journal of Technology Assessment in Health Care 1990;**6**(03):480–8.

5 Sackett D, Ellis J, Mulligan I, et al. Inpatient general medicine is evidence based. The Lancet 1995;**346**(8972):407–10.

6 Runciman WB, Hunt TD, Hannaford NA, et al. CareTrack: assessing the appropriateness of health care delivery in Australia. Medical Journal of Australia 2012;**197**(10):549.

7 Macnaughton J. Anecdote in clinical practice. In: Greenhalgh T, Hurwitz B, eds. *Narrative based medicine: dialogue and discourse in clinical practice.* London: BMJ Publications, 1998.

8 Greenhalgh T. Narrative based medicine: narrative based medicine in an evidence based world. BMJ: British Medical Journal 1999;**318**(7179):323.

9 Greenhalgh T. Intuition and evidence – uneasy bedfellows? The British Journal of General Practice 2002;**52**(478):395.

10 Mori R, Lakhanpaul M, Verrier-Jones K. Guidelines: diagnosis and management of urinary tract infection in children: summary of NICE guidance. BMJ: British Medical Journal 2007;**335**(7616):395.

11 Mulrow CD. Rationale for systematic reviews. BMJ: British Medical Journal 1994;**309**(6954):597.

12 van Helmont JA. *Oriatrike, or physick refined: the common errors therein refuted and the whole art reformed and rectified.* London: Lodowick-Loyd, 1662.

13 Swinglehurst DA. Information needs of United Kingdom primary care clinicians. Health Information & Libraries Journal 2005;**22**(3):196–204.
14 Smith R. Where is the wisdom … ? BMJ: British Medical Journal 1991; **303**(6806):798.
15 Straus SE, Richardson WS, Glasziou P, et al. *Evidence-based medicine: how to practice and teach EBM* (Fourth Edition). Edinburgh: Churchill Livingstone, 2010.

Chapter 2 **Searching the literature**

Evidence is accumulating faster than ever before, and staying current is essential for quality patient care.

Studies and reviews of studies of doctors' information-seeking behaviour confirm that textbooks and personal contacts continue to be the most favoured sources for clinical information, followed by journal articles (see, e.g. [1]). Use of the Internet as an information resource has increased dramatically in recent years, especially via PubMed/Medline, but the sophistication of searching and the efficiency in finding answers has not grown apace. Indeed, ask any medical librarian and you will hear tales of important clinical questions being addressed using unsystematic Google searches. While the need of healthcare professionals for information of the best quality has never been greater, barriers abound: lack of time, lack of facilities, lack of searching skills, lack of motivation and (perhaps worst of all) information overload [2].

The medical literature is far more of a jungle today than it was when the first edition of this book was published in 1996. The volume and complexity of published literature has grown: Medline alone has over 20 million references. While Medline is the flagship database for journal articles in the health sciences, it is a very conservative resource, slow to pick up new journals or journals published outside the USA, so there are many thousands of high-quality papers that may be available via other databases but are not included in Medline's 20 million. The proliferation of databases makes the information jungle that much more confusing, especially because each database covers its own range of journals and each has its own particular search protocols. How will you cope?

There is hope: in the past decade, the information 'jungle' has been tamed by means of information highways and high-speed transit systems. Knowing

How to Read a Paper: The Basics of Evidence-Based Medicine, Fifth Edition. Trisha Greenhalgh.
© 2014 John Wiley & Sons, Ltd. Published 2014 by John Wiley & Sons, Ltd.

how to access these navigational wonders will save you time and improve your ability to find the best evidence. The purpose of this chapter is not to teach you to become an expert searcher but rather to help you recognise the kinds of resources that are available, choose intelligently among them and put them to work directly.

What are you looking for?

A searcher may approach medical (and, more broadly, health science) literature for three broad purposes:

- Informally, almost recreationally, browsing to keep current and to satisfy our intrinsic curiosity;
- Focused, looking for answers, perhaps related to questions that have occurred in clinic or that arise from individual patients and their questions;
- Surveying the existing literature, perhaps before embarking on a research project.

Each approach involves searching in a very different way.

Browsing has an element of serendipity about it. In the old days, we would pick up our favourite journal and follow where our fancy took us. And if our fancy was informed with a few tools to help us discriminate the quality of papers we found, so much the better. These days, we can make use of new tools to help us with our browsing. We can browse electronic journals just as easily as paper journals; we can use alerting services to let us know when a new issue has been published and even tell us if articles matching our interest profile are in that issue. We can have Rich Site Summary (RSS) feeds of articles from particular journals or on particular topics sent to our e-mail addresses or our i-Phones or personal blogs, and we can participate in Twitter exchanges related to newly published papers. Almost every journal has links from its home page allowing at least one of these social networking services. These technologies are changing continuously. Those of us who have been faced with deluges of new off-prints, photocopies and journal issues we have been meaning to read will be happy to learn that we can create the same chaos electronically. That is what browsing serendipitously is all about, and it is a joy we should never lose, in whatever medium our literature may be published.

Looking for answers implies a much more focused approach, a search for an answer we can trust to apply directly to the care of a patient. When we find that trustworthy information, it is OK to stop looking – we don't need to beat the bush for absolutely every study that may have addressed this topic. This kind of query is increasingly well served by new synthesised information sources whose goal is to support evidence-based care and the transfer of research findings into practice. This is discussed further here.

Surveying the literature – preparing a detailed, broad-based and thoughtful literature review, for example, when writing an essay for an assignment or an article for publication – involves an entirely different process. The purpose here is less to influence patient care directly than to identify the existing body of research that has addressed a problem and clarify the gaps in knowledge that require further research. For this kind of searching, a strong knowledge of information resources and skill in searching them are fundamental. A simple PubMed search will not suffice. Multiple relevant databases need to be searched systematically, and citation chaining (see subsequent text) needs to be employed to assure that no stone has been left unturned. If this is your goal, you *must* consult with an information professional (health librarian, clinical informationist, etc.).

Levels upon levels of evidence

The term *level of evidence* refers to what degree that information can be trusted, based on study design. Traditionally, and considering the commonest type of question (relating to therapy), levels of evidence are represented as a pyramid with systematic reviews positioned grandly at the top, followed by well-designed randomised controlled trials, then observational studies such as cohort studies or case–control studies, with case studies, bench (laboratory) studies and 'expert opinion' somewhere near the bottom (Figure 2.1). This traditional hierarchy is described in more detail in section 'The traditional hierarchy of evidence'.

My librarian colleagues, who are often keen on synthesised evidence and technical resources for decision support, remind me of a rival pyramid, with computerised decision support systems at the top, above evidence-based practice guidelines, followed by systematic review synopses, with standard systematic reviews beneath these, and so on [3].

Whether we think in terms of the first (traditional) evidence pyramid or the second (more contemporary) one, the message is clear: all evidence, all information, is not necessarily equivalent. We need to keep a sharp eye out for the believability of whatever information we find, wherever we find it.

Synthesised sources: systems, summaries and syntheses

Information resources synthesised from primary studies constitute a very high level of evidence indeed. These resources exist to help translate research into practice and inform clinician and patient decision-making. This kind of

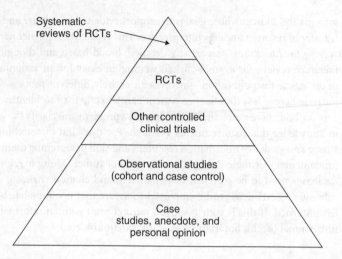

Figure 2.1 A simple hierarchy of evidence for assessing the quality of trial design in therapy studies.

evidence is relatively new (at least, compared to traditional primary research studies, which have been with us for centuries), but their use is expected to grow considerably as they become better known.

Systematic reviews are perhaps the oldest and best known of the synthesised sources, having started in the 1980s under the inspiration of Archie Cochrane, who bemoaned the multiplicity of individual clinical trials whose information failed to provide clear messages for practice. The original efforts to search broadly for clinical trials on a topic and pool their results statistically grew into the Cochrane Library in the mid-1990s; Cochrane Reviews became the gold standard for systematic reviews and the Cochrane Collaboration the premier force for developing and improving review methodology [4].

There are many advantages to systematic reviews and a few cautions. On the plus side, systematic reviews are relatively easy to interpret. The systematic selection and appraisal of the primary studies according to an approved protocol means that bias is minimised. Smaller studies, which are all too common in some topic areas, may show a trend towards positive impact but lack statistical significance. But when data from several small studies are summed mathematically in a process called *meta-analysis*, the combined data may produce a statistically significant finding (see section 'Meta-analysis for the non-statistician'). Systematic reviews can help resolve contradictory findings among different studies on the same question. If the systematic review has been properly conducted, the results are likely to be robust and generalisable. On the negative side, systematic reviews can replicate and magnify flaws in the original studies (e.g. if all the primary studies considered a drug at sub-therapeutic dose, the overall – misleading – conclusion may be that the drug has 'no effect'). Cochrane Reviews can be a daunting read, but here's a tip. The bulk of a Cochrane Review consists of methodological discussion: the gist of it can be gleaned by jumping to the 'Plain Language Summary', always to be found directly following the abstract. Alternatively, you can gain a quick and accurate summary by looking at the pictures – especially something called a *forest plot*, which graphically displays the results of each of the primary studies along with the combined result. Chapter 9 explains systematic reviews in more detail.

Cochrane Reviews are only published electronically, but other systematic reviews appear throughout the clinical literature. They are most easily accessed via the Cochrane Library, which publishes Cochrane Reviews, DARE (Database of Abstracts of Reviews of Effects, listed in Cochrane Library as 'Other reviews'), and a database of Health Technology Assessments (HTAs). DARE provides not only a bibliography of systematic reviews but also a critical appraisal of most of the reviews included, making this a 'pre-appraised source' for systematic reviews. HTAs are essentially systematic reviews but range further to consider economic and policy implications of drugs, technologies and health systems. All may be searched relatively simply and simultaneously via the Cochrane Library.

In the past, Cochrane Reviews focused mainly on questions of therapy (see Chapter 6) or prevention, but since 2008, considerable effort has gone into producing systematic reviews of diagnostic tests (see Chapter 8).

Point-of-care resources are rather like electronic textbooks or detailed clinical handbooks, but explicitly evidence-based, continuously updated and designed to be user-friendly – perhaps, the textbook of the future. Three popular ones are *Clinical Evidence, DynaMed* and *American College of Physicians Physicians' Information and Education Resource* (*ACP PIER*). All of these aspire to be firmly evidence-based, peer-reviewed, revised regularly and with links to the primary research incorporated into their recommendations.

- *Clinical Evidence* (http://clinicalevidence.bmj.com), a British resource, draws on systematic reviews to provide very quick information, especially on the comparative value of tests and interventions. Reviews are organised into sections, such as Child Health or Skin Disorders; or you can search them by keyword (e.g. 'asthma') or by a full review list. The opening page of a chapter lists questions about the effectiveness of various interventions and flags using gold, white or red medallions to indicate whether the evidence for these is positive, equivocal or negative.
- *DynaMed* (http://www.ebscohost.com/dynamed/), produced in the USA, is rather more like a handbook with chapters covering a wide variety of disorders, but with summaries of clinical research, levels of evidence and

links to the primary articles. It covers causes and risks, complications and associated conditions (including differential diagnosis), what to look for in the history and physical examination, what diagnostic tests to do, prognosis, treatment, prevention and screening and links to patient information handouts. You can search very simply for the condition: the results include links to other chapters about similar conditions. This is a proprietary resource (i.e. you generally have to pay for it), although it may be provided free to those who offer to write a chapter themselves!

- *ACP PIER* (*American College of Physicians Physicians' Information and Education Resource* – http://pier.acponline.org) is another US source. It uses the standard format of broad recommendation, specific recommendation, rationale and evidence, ACP PIER covers prevention, screening, diagnosis, consultation, hospitalization, drug and non-drug treatments and follow-up. Links to the primary literature are provided and a 'Patient information' tab provides links to websites patients would find helpful and authoritative.

Both PIER and DynaMed have applications facilitating use on personal digital assistants (PDAs) or other hand-held devices, which improve their bedside usability for patient care.

New point-of-care resources are continually emerging, so it is very much a matter of individual preference which you use. The three listed were chosen because they are peer-reviewed, regularly updated and directly linked to the primary evidence.

Practice Guidelines, covered in detail in Chapter 10, are 'systematically developed statements to assist practitioner and patient decisions about appropriate healthcare for specific clinical circumstances' [5]. In a good guideline, the scientific evidence is assembled systematically, the panel developing the guideline includes representatives from all relevant disciplines, including patients, and the recommendations are explicitly linked to the evidence from which they are derived [6]. Guidelines are a summarised form of evidence, very high on the hierarchy of pre-appraised resources, but the initial purpose of the guideline should always be kept in mind: guidelines for different settings and different purposes can be based on the same evidence but come out with different recommendations.

Guidelines are readily available from a variety of sources, including the following.

- *National Guideline Clearinghouse* (http://www.guideline.gov/) is an initiative of the Agency for Healthcare Research and Quality (AHRQ), U.S. Department of Health and Human Services. Although a government-funded US database, National Geographic Channel (NGC) is international in content. An advantage of this resource is that different guidelines purporting to cover the same topic can be directly compared on all points, from levels of evidence to recommendations. All guidelines must be current and revised every 5 years.

- *National Institute for Health and Care Excellence* (*NICE*, http://www.nice .org.uk/) is a UK-government-funded agency responsible for developing evidence-based guidelines and other evidence summaries to support national health policy. NICE Clinical Knowledge Summaries (http://cks .nice.org.uk) are designed especially for those working in primary healthcare.

A straightforward and popular way to search practice guidelines is via TRIP (Turning Research into Practice, http://www.tripdatabase.com), a federated search engine discussed subsequently. For guidelines, look in the box panel to the right of the screen following a simple search: a heading 'guidelines' appears, with subheadings for Australian and New Zealand, Canadian, UK, USA and Other, and a number indicting the number of guidelines found on that topic. NICE and National Guideline Clearinghouse are included among the guidelines searched.

Pre-appraised sources: synopses of systematic reviews and primary studies

If your topic is more circumscribed than those covered in the synthesised or summary sources we have explored, or if you are simply browsing to keep current with the literature, consider one of the pre-appraised sources as a means of navigating through those millions of articles in our information jungle. The most common format is the digest of clinical research articles gleaned from core journals and deemed to provide important information for patient care: *Evidence-Based Medicine, ACP Journal Club, Evidence-Based Mental Health, POEMS (Patient-Oriented Evidence that Matters)*. Some are free, some are available through institutions or memberships or private sub-scription. All of them have a format that includes a structured abstract and a brief critical appraisal of the article's content. Studies included may be single studies or systematic reviews. Each is considered a pre-appraised source, and critical appraisal aside, simple inclusion has implications for the perceived quality and importance of the original article.

All of these sources may be considered as small databases of select studies, which may be searched by keyword. Other selected journal article services, such as Evidence Updates, provide abstracts plus an indication of level of interest each article might hold for particular disciplines.

DARE was mentioned as a pre-appraised source for systematic reviews other than Cochrane Reviews, in that it provides an augmented abstract and a brief critical appraisal for most systematic reviews in its database.

Another source that is considered pre-appraised, although it contains no appraisals, is the *Central Register of Controlled Trials*, also part of the Cochrane Library. 'Central' is a bibliography of studies included in Cochrane Reviews, as well as in new studies on similar topics, maintained by the various Cochrane Review Groups. DARE, Central, the Cochrane Database of Systematic Reviews, the HTA database and the NHS Economic Evaluation Database – which also includes critically appraised summaries of studies – may all be searched simultaneously in the Cochrane Library.

Specialised resources

Specialised information sources, organised (as the name implies) to assist the specialist doctor in a particular field, are often also useful for generalists, specialist nurses and primary care clinicians. Most professional associations maintain excellent websites with practice guidelines, journal links and other useful information resources; most require membership in the association to access educational and practice materials. Three notable examples that are available for a fee are Global Infectious Diseases and Epidemiology Network (GIDEON), Psychiatry Online and CardioSource.

- *GIDEON (Global Infectious Diseases and Epidemiology Network*, http://www.gideononline.com/) is an evidence-based programme that assists with diagnosis and treatment of communicable diseases. In addition, GIDEON tracks incidence and prevalence of diseases worldwide and includes the spectrum covered by antibiotic agents.
- *Psychiatry Online* (http://www.psychiatryonline.com/) is a compendium of core textbooks (including Diagnostic and Statistical Manual of Mental Disorders fifth edition (DSM V)), psychiatry journals and practice guidelines of the American Psychiatric Association, produced by the American Psychiatric Press.
- *CardioSource* (http://www.cardiosource.com) is produced by the American College of Cardiology. It includes guidelines, journal and textbook links, 'clinical collections' of articles and educational materials on topics such as cholesterol management and atrial fibrillation, and an excellent clinical trials registry for all trials relating to cardiovascular disease, whether ongoing or completed.

These three are only examples. Whatever your specialty (or specialist topic), there will usually be a similar resource maintained by a professional society. Ask a librarian or clinical informaticist to help you find the relevant one!

Primary studies – tackling the jungle

Whether through habit or through lack of familiarity with all the useful synthesised, summarised or pre-appraised sources described earlier, most health practitioners still prefer a basic search of Medline/PubMed to answer their clinical information needs. Some simply prefer to assess the primary literature for themselves, without thumbnail critical appraisals or incorporation into larger disease management chapters. I still advise you to go for the secondary sources described in sections 'Levels upon levels of evidence', 'Synthesised sources: systems, summaries and syntheses' and 'Pre-appraised sources: synopses of systematic reviews and primary studies', but if you would like to go direct to the primary studies, this section is for you.

Primary sources can be found in a variety of ways. You could look at the reference lists and hyperlinks from the secondary sources described. You could identify them from journals – for example, via RSS feeds, table-of-contents services or more focused topical information services. And you could search databases such as PubMed/Medline, EMBASE, PASCAL, Cochrane Library, CINAHL (Cumulated Index of Nursing and Allied Health Literature), Biosis Previews, Web of Science, Scopus or Google or Google Scholar. I consider these one by one here.

PubMed is the most frequently accessed Internet resource for most physicians and health professionals worldwide, probably because it is free and well-known. Most people opt for the basic PubMed search, using two or three search text words at best – and characteristically turning up hundreds or thousands of references, of which they look at only the first couple of screens. This is certainly not the most efficient way to search, but it is the reality of how most people *do* search [7]. Interestingly, when just one or two more search terms are added, the efficiency of a basic PubMed search improves substantially [7].

Simple tools that are part of the Medline search engine can be used to help focus a search and produce better results for a basic search, but they are rarely used by medical students or doctors. One such tool is the '*limit*' function, allowing restrictions to such generic topics as gender, age group or study design; to language or to core clinical journals. The advanced search function on PubMed incorporates these limits into a single search page. Next time you are on the PubMed website with some time to spare, play with these tools and see how easily they can sharpen your search.

'*Clinical queries*', an option provided in the left-hand panel of the basic PubMed screen or at the bottom of the advanced search screen, superimposes on the search a filter based on optimum study designs for best evidence, depending on the domain of the question and the degree to which one wishes to focus the question. For example, if you were searching for a therapy study for hypercholesterolaemia, the clinical query for therapy/narrow and specific would be rendered as '(hypercholesterolaemia) AND (randomised controlled trial [Publication Type] OR (randomised [Title/Abstract] AND controlled [Title/Abstract] AND trial [Title/Abstract]))'. In this instance, the search might need further limits or perhaps the addition of a second term, such as a specific drug, because the result is over 2000 postings.

Citation chaining (or, to use its alternative term, *citation tracking*) provides another means of following a topic. Let's say that, following your interest in hypercholesterolaemia, you wish to follow up a classic primary research study, the West of Scotland Coronary Prevention Study, originally published in the 1990s [8]. In your PubMed search, you found a study in the New England Journal of Medicine in 2007 that described a 20-year follow-up [9], but you now wonder if there has been anything further. The databases Web of Science, comprising Science Citation Index, Social Sciences Citation Index and the Arts and Humanities Citation Index online, provide a cited reference search feature. Entering the author's name (in this case I. Ford) and the year of publication (2007), we can trace the specific article, and find that several dozen articles published since have cited it in their reference lists. Citation searching can give a crude indication of the relative importance of a study, based on the number of times it has been cited (bearing in mind that one sometimes cites a paper when emphasising how bad it is!). A very simple (but somewhat less accurate) way of citation chaining is to use Google Scholar: simply put the article's title into this search engine and when you have found it, select 'citations'.

Google Scholar, a very broad-based web browser, is increasingly popular and extremely handy, accessible as it is from the Google toolbar. For an obscure topic, Google Scholar can be an excellent resource on which to fall back, as it will identify papers that are listed on PubMed as well as those that aren't. Unfortunately, there are no quality filters (such as clinical queries), no limits (such as gender or age), so a search on a widely researched topic will tend to turn up a long list of hits that you have no alternative but to wade through.

One-stop shopping: federated search engines

Perhaps the simplest and most efficient answer for most clinicians searching for information for patient care is a federated search engine such as TRIP, http://www.tripdatabase.com/, which searches multiple resources simultaneously and has the advantage of being free.

TRIP has a truly primitive search engine, but it searches synthesised sources (systematic reviews including Cochrane Reviews), summarised sources (including practice guidelines from North America, Europe, Australia/New Zealand and elsewhere, as well as electronic textbooks) and pre-appraised sources (such as the journals *Evidence-Based Medicine* and *Evidence-Based Mental Health*), as well as searching all clinical query domains in PubMed simultaneously. Moreover, searches can be limited by discipline, such as Paediatrics or Surgery, helping both to focus a search and eliminate clearly irrelevant results and acknowledging the tendency of medical specialists to (rightly or wrongly) prefer the literature in their own journals. Given that most clinicians favour very simple searches, a TRIP search may well get you the maximum bang for your buck.

Asking for help and asking around

If a librarian fractured her wrist, she would have no hesitation in seeking out a physician. Similarly, a healthcare professional doesn't need to cope with the literature alone. Health librarians are readily available in universities, hospitals, government departments and agencies and professional societies. They know the databases available, they know the complexities of searching, they know the literature (even complex government documents and obscure data sets), and they usually know just enough about the topic to have an idea of what you are looking for and levels of evidence that are likely to be found. When one librarian can't find an answer, there are colleagues with whom he can and will consult, locally, nationally and internationally. Librarians of the 21st century are exceptionally well networked!

Asking people you know yourself or know about has its advantages. Experts in the field are often aware of unpublished research or reports commissioned by government or other agencies – notoriously hard-to-find 'grey' or 'fugitive' literature that is not indexed in any source. An international organised information-sharing organisation CHAIN (Contact, Help, Advice and Information Network, http://chain.ulcc.ac.uk/chain) provides a useful online network for people working in health and social care who wish to share information. CHAIN can be joined for free and once a member, you can pitch in a question and target it to a designated group of specialists.

In a field as overwhelming and complex as health information, asking colleagues and people you trust has always been a preferred source for information. In the early days of evidence-based medicine (EBM), asking around was seen as unsystematic and 'biased'. It remains true that asking around is insufficient for a search for evidence, but in the light of the ability of experts to locate obscure literature, can any search really be considered complete with-out it?

Online tutorials for effective searching

Many universities and other educational institutions now provide self-study tutorials, which you can access via computer – either on an intranet (for members of the university only) or the Internet (accessible to everyone). Here are some I found when revising this chapter for the fifth edition. Note that as with all Internet-based sources, some sites will move or close down, so I apologise in advance if you find a dead link:

- *'Finding the Evidence'* from the University of Oxford's Centre for Evidence-Based Medicine. Some brief advice on searching key databases but relatively little in the way of teaching you how to do it. Perhaps best for those who have already been on a course and want to refresh their memory. http://www.cebm.net/index.aspx?o=1038.
- *'PubMed – Searching Medical Literature'* from the Library at Georgia State University. As the title implies, this is limited to PubMed but offers some advanced tricks such as how to customise the PubMed interface to suit your personal needs. http://research.library.gsu.edu/pubmed.
- *'PubMed Tutorial'* from PubMed itself. Offers an overview of what PubMed does and doesn't do, as well as some exercises to get used to it. http://www.nlm.nih.gov/bsd/disted/pubmedtutorial/.

There are many other similar tutorials accessible free on the Internet, but few of them cover much beyond searching for primary studies and systematic reviews in PubMed and the Cochrane Library. I hope that by the time the next edition of this book is due, someone will have redressed this bias and developed tutorials on how to access the full range of summaries, syntheses and pre-appraised sources I described in earlier sections.

References

1 Davies K. The information seeking behaviour of doctors: a review of the evidence. Health Information & Libraries Journal 2007;**24**(2):78–94.
2 Fourie I. Learning from research on the information behaviour of healthcare pro-fessionals: a review of the literature 2004–2008 with a focus on emotion. Health Information & Libraries Journal 2009;**26**(3):171–86.
3 DiCenso A, Bayley L, Haynes R. ACP Journal Club. Editorial: accessing preappraised evidence: fine-tuning the 5S model into a 6S model. Annals of Internal Medicine 2009;**151**(6):JC3.
4 Levin A. The Cochrane collaboration. Annals of Internal Medicine 2001;**135**(4): 309–12.

5 Field MJ, Lohr KN. *Clinical practice guidelines: directions for a new program.* Washington, DC: National Academy Press, 1990.

6 Grimshaw J, Freemantle N, Wallace S, et al. Developing and implementing clinical practice guidelines. Quality in Health Care 1995;**4**(1):55.

7 Hoogendam A, Stalenhoef AF, de Vries Robbé PF, et al. Answers to questions posed during daily patient care are more likely to be answered by UpToDate than PubMed. Journal of Medical Internet Research 2008;**10**(4):e29.

8 Shepherd J, Cobbe SM, Ford I, et al. Prevention of coronary heart disease with pravastatin in men with hypercholesterolemia. The New England Journal of Medicine 1995;**333**(20):1301–7 doi: 10.1056/nejm199511163332001.

9 Ford I, Murray H, Packard CJ, et al. Long-term follow-up of the West of Scotland Coronary Prevention Study. The New England Journal of Medicine 2007;**357**(15):1477–86 doi: 10.1056/NEJMoa065994.

Chapter 3 Getting your bearings: what is this paper about?

The science of 'trashing' papers

It usually comes as a surprise to students to learn that some (the purists would say up to 99% of) published articles belong in the bin, and should certainly not be used to inform practice. In 1979, the editor of the British Medical Journal, Dr Stephen Lock, wrote 'Few things are more dispiriting to a medical editor than having to reject a paper based on a good idea but with irremediable flaws in the methods used'. Fifteen years later, Altman was still claiming that only 1% of medical research was free of methodological flaws [1]; and more recently he confirmed that serious and fundamental flaws commonly occur even in papers published in 'quality' journals [2]. Box 3.1 shows the main flaws that lead to papers being rejected (and which are present to some degree in many that end up published).

Most papers appearing in medical journals these days are presented more or less in standard Introduction, Methods, Research and Discussion (IMRAD) format: Introduction (*why* the authors decided to do this particular piece of research), Methods (*how* they did it, and how they chose to analyse their results), Results (*what* they found) and Discussion (what they think the results *mean*). If you are deciding whether a paper is worth reading, you should do so on the design of the methods section, and not on the interest value of the hypothesis, the nature or potential impact of the results or the speculation in the discussion.

Conversely, bad science is bad science regardless of whether the study addressed an important clinical issue, whether the results are 'statistically significant' (see section 'Probability and confidence'), whether things changed in the direction you would have liked them to and whether the findings promise immeasurable benefits for patients or savings for the

How to Read a Paper: The Basics of Evidence-Based Medicine, Fifth Edition. Trisha Greenhalgh.
© 2014 John Wiley & Sons, Ltd. Published 2014 by John Wiley & Sons, Ltd.

Box 3.1 Common reasons why papers are rejected for publication

1. The study did not address an important scientific issue (see section 'Three preliminary questions to get your bearings').
2. The study was not original – that is someone else has already performed the same or a similar study (see section 'Was the study original?').
3. The study did not actually test the authors' hypothesis (see section 'Three preliminary questions to get your bearings').
4. A different study design should have been used (see section 'Randomised controlled trials').
5. Practical difficulties (e.g. in recruiting participants) led the authors to compromise on the original study protocol (see section 'Was the design of the study sensible?').
6. The sample size was too small (see section 'Were preliminary statistical questions addressed?').
7. The study was uncontrolled or inadequately controlled (see section 'Was systematic bias avoided or minimised?').
8. The statistical analysis was incorrect or inappropriate (see Chapter 5).
9. The authors have drawn unjustified conclusions from their data.
10. There is a significant conflict of interest (e.g. one of the authors, or a sponsor, might benefit financially from the publication of the paper and insufficient safeguards were seen to be in place to guard against bias).
11. The paper is so badly written that it is incomprehensible.

---

health service. Strictly speaking, *if you are going to trash a paper, you should do so before you even look at the results.*

It is much easier to pick holes in other people's work than to do a methodologically perfect piece of research oneself. When I teach critical appraisal, there is usually someone in the group who finds it profoundly discourteous to criticise research projects into which dedicated scientists have put the best years of their lives. On a more pragmatic note, there may be good practical reasons why the authors of the study have not performed a perfect study, and they know as well as you do that their work would have been more scientifically valid if this or that (anticipated or unanticipated) difficulty had not arisen during the course of the study.

Most good scientific journals send papers out to a referee for comments on their scientific validity, originality and importance before deciding whether to publish them. This process is known as *peer review*, and much has been written about it [3]. Common defects picked up by referees are listed in Box 3.1.

The assessment of methodological quality (critical appraisal) has been covered in detail in the widely cited series led by Gordon Guyatt, 'Users' Guides to the Medical Literature' (for the full list and links to the free full text of most of them, see JAMA Evidence http://www.cche.net/usersguides/main.asp). The structured guides produced by these authors on how to read papers on therapy, diagnosis, screening, prognosis, causation, quality of care, economic analysis, systematic review, qualitative research and so on are regarded by many as the definitive checklists for critical appraisal. Appendix 1 lists some simpler checklists I have derived from the Users' Guides and the other sources cited at the end of this chapter, together with some ideas of my own. If you are an experienced journal reader, these checklists will be largely self-explanatory. But if you still have difficulty getting started when looking at a medical paper, try asking the preliminary questions in the next section.

Three preliminary questions to get your bearings

Question One: What was the research question – and why was the study needed?
The introductory sentence of a research paper should state, in a nutshell, what the background to the research is. For example, 'Grommet insertion is a common procedure in children, and it has been suggested that not all operations are clinically necessary'. This statement should be followed by a brief review of the published literature, for example, 'Gupta and Brown's prospective survey of grommet insertions demonstrated that … '. It is irritatingly common for authors to forget to place their research in context, as the background to the problem is usually clear as daylight to them by the time they reach the writing-up stage.

Unless it has already been covered in the introduction, the methods section of the paper should state clearly the research question and/or the hypothesis that the authors have decided to test. For example: 'This study aimed to determine whether day case hernia surgery was safer and more acceptable to patients than the standard inpatient procedure'.

You may find that the research question has inadvertently been omitted, or, more commonly, that the information is buried somewhere mid-paragraph. If the main research hypothesis is presented in the negative (which it usually is), such as 'The addition of metformin to maximal dose sulphonylurea therapy will not improve the control of Type 2 diabetes', it is known as a *null* hypothesis. The authors of a study rarely actually *believe* their null hypothesis when they embark on their research. Being human, they have usually set out to demonstrate a difference between the two arms of their study. But the way scientists do this is to say 'let's *assume* there's no difference; now let's try to disprove that theory'. If you adhere to the teachings of Popper, this *hypotheticodeductive* approach (setting up falsifiable hypotheses that you then proceed to test) is the very essence of the scientific method [4].

If you have not discovered what the authors' research question was by the time you are halfway through the methods section, you may find it in the first paragraph of the discussion. Remember, however, that not all research studies (even good ones) are set up to test a single definitive hypothesis. *Qualitative* research studies, which (so long as they are well-designed and well-conducted) are as valid and as necessary as the more conventional quantitative studies, aim to look at particular issues in a broad, open-ended way in order to illuminate issues; generate or modify hypotheses and prioritise areas to investigate. This type of research is discussed further in Chapter 12. Even quantitative research (which most of the rest of this book is about) is now seen as more than hypothesis-testing. As section 'Probability and confidence' argues, it is strictly preferable to talk about evaluating the *strength* of evidence around a particular issue than about proving or disproving hypotheses.

Question Two: What was the research design?

First, decide whether the paper describes a primary or secondary study. Primary studies report research first-hand, while secondary studies attempt to summarise and draw conclusions from primary studies. Primary studies (sometimes known as *empirical studies*) are the stuff of most published research in medical journals, and usually fall into one of three categories:

- *Laboratory experiments*, in which a manoeuvre is performed on an animal or a volunteer in artificial and controlled surroundings;
- *Clinical trials*, a form of experiment in which an intervention – either simple (such as a drug; see Chapter 6) or complex (such as an educational programme; see Chapter 7) – is offered to a group of participants (i.e. the patients included in the trial) who are then followed up to see what happens to them;
- *Surveys*, in which something is measured in a group of participants (patients, health professionals or some other sample of individuals). Questionnaire surveys (Chapter 13) measure people's opinions, attitudes and self-reported behaviours; or
- *Organisational case studies*, in which the researcher tells a story that tries to capture the complexity of a change effort (e.g. an attempt to implement evidence; Chapter 14).

The commoner types of clinical trials and surveys are discussed in the later sections of this chapter. Make sure you understand any jargon used in describing the study design (see Table 3.1).

Table 3.1 Terms used to describe design features of clinical research studies

Term	Meaning
Parallel group comparison	Each group receives a different treatment, with both groups being entered at the same time. In this case, results are analysed by comparing groups.
Paired (or matched) comparison	Participants receiving different treatments are matched to balance potential confounding variables such as age and sex. Results are analysed in terms of differences between participant pairs.
Within-participant comparison	Participants are assessed before and after an intervention and results analysed in terms of within-participant changes.
Single-blind	Participants did not know which treatment they were receiving.
Double-blind	Neither did the investigators.
Crossover	Each participant received both the intervention and control treatments (in random order), often separated by a *washout* period on no treatment.
Placebo-controlled	Control participants receive a placebo (inactive pill) that should look and taste the same as the active pill. Placebo (sham) operations may also be used in trials of surgery.
Factorial design	A study that permits investigation of the effects (both separately and combined) of more than one independent variable on a given outcome (e.g. a 2 × 2 factorial design tested the effects of placebo, aspirin alone, streptokinase alone or aspirin + streptokinase in acute heart attack [5]).

Secondary research is composed of the following
- *Overviews*, which are considered in Chapter 9, may be divided into
  (a) *(non-systematic) reviews*, which summarise primary studies;
  (b) *systematic reviews*, which do this using a rigorous, transparent and auditable (i.e. checkable) method;
  (c) *meta-analyses*, which integrate the numerical data from more than one study;
- *Guidelines*, which are considered in Chapter 10, draw conclusions from primary studies about how clinicians should be behaving;
- *Decision analyses*, which are not discussed in detail in this book but are covered elsewhere [6], use the results of primary studies to generate probability trees to be used by both health professionals and patients in making choices about clinical management;

- *Economic analyses*, which are considered briefly in Chapter 12 and in more detail elsewhere [7], use the results of primary studies to say whether a particular course of action is a good use of resources.

Question Three: Was the research design appropriate to the question?

Examples of the sort of questions that can reasonably be answered by different types of primary research study are given in the sections that follow. One question that frequently cries out to be asked is this: was a randomised controlled trial (RCT) (see section 'Randomised controlled trials') the best method of addressing this particular research question, and if the study was not an RCT, should it have been? Before you jump to any conclusions, decide what broad field of research the study covers (see Box 3.2). Once you have done this, ask whether the study design was appropriate to this question. For more help on this task (which people often find difficult until they get the hang of it) see the Oxford Centre for Evidence-Based Medicine (EBM) website (www.cebm.ox.ac.uk).

Box 3.2 Broad fields of research

Most quantitative studies are concerned with one or more of the following:

- *Therapy*: testing the efficacy of drug treatments, surgical procedures, alternative methods of service delivery or other interventions. Preferred study design is randomised controlled trial (see section 'Randomised controlled trials' and Chapters 6 and 7).
- *Diagnosis*: demonstrating whether a new diagnostic test is valid (can we trust it?) and reliable (would we get the same results every time?). Preferred study design is cross-sectional survey (see section 'Cross-sectional surveys' and Chapter 8).
- *Screening*: demonstrating the value of tests that can be applied to large populations and that pick up disease at a pre-symptomatic stage. Preferred study design is cross-sectional survey (see section 'Cross-sectional surveys' and Chapter 8).
- *Prognosis*: determining what is likely to happen to someone whose disease is picked up at an early stage. Preferred study design is longitudinal survey (see section 'Cross-sectional surveys').
- *Causation*: determining whether a putative harmful agent, such as environmental pollution, is related to the development of illness. Preferred study design is cohort or case–control study, depending on how rare the disease is (see sections 'Cross-sectional surveys' and 'Case reports'), but case reports

---

(see section 'The traditional hierarchy of evidence') may also provide crucial information.

- *Psychometric studies*: measuring attitudes, beliefs or preferences, often about the nature of illness or its treatment.

Qualitative studies are discussed in Chapter 12.

Randomised controlled trials

In an RCT, participants in the trial are randomly allocated by a process equivalent to the flip of a coin to either one intervention (such as a drug treatment) or another (such as placebo treatment – or more commonly, best current therapy). Both groups are followed up for a pre-specified time period and analysed in terms of specific outcomes defined at the outset of the study (e.g. death, heart attack, and serum cholesterol level). Because, *on average*, the groups are identical apart from the intervention, any differences in outcome are, in theory, attributable to the intervention. In reality, however, not every RCT is a bowl of cherries.

Some papers that report trials comparing an intervention with a control group are not, in fact, randomised trials at all. The terminology for these is *other controlled clinical trials* – a term used to describe comparative studies in which participants were allocated to intervention or control groups in a non-random manner. This situation may arise, for example, when random allocation would be impossible, impractical or unethical – for example, when patients on ward A receive one diet while those on ward B receive a different diet. (Although this design is inferior to the RCT, it is much easier to execute, and was used successfully a century ago to demonstrate the benefit of brown rice over white rice in the treatment of beriberi [8].) The problems of non-random allocation are discussed further in section 'Was systematic bias avoided or minimised?' in relation to determining whether the two groups in a trial can reasonably be compared with one another on a statistical level.

Some trials count as a sort of halfway house between true randomised trials and non-randomised trials. In these, randomisation is not performed truly at random (e.g. using sequentially numbered sealed envelopes each with a computer-generated random number inside), but by some method that allows the clinician to know which group the patient would be in *before he or she makes a definitive decision to randomise the patient*. This allows subtle biases to creep in, as the clinician might be more (or less) likely to enter a particular patient into the trial if he or she believed that this individual would get active treatment. In particular, patients with more severe disease may be subconsciously withheld from the placebo arm of the trial. Examples of unacceptable methods include randomisation by last digit of date of birth (even numbers to group A, odds to group B), toss of a coin (heads to group A, tails to group B), sequential allocation (patient A to group 1; patient B to group 2, etc.) and date seen in clinic (all patients seen this week to group A; all those seen next week to group 2, etc.) (Box 3.3) [9, 10].

Listed here are examples of clinical questions that would be best answered by an RCT, but note also the examples in the later sections of this chapter of situations where other types of studies could or must be used instead.

- Is this drug better than a placebo or a different drug for a particular disease?
- Is a new surgical procedure better than the currently favoured practice?
- Is an online decision support algorithm better than verbal advice in helping patients make informed choices about the treatment options for a particular condition?
- Will changing from a diet high in saturated fats to one high in polyunsaturated fats significantly affect serum cholesterol levels?

RCTs are often said to be the gold standard in medical research. Up to a point, this is true (see section 'The traditional hierarchy of evidence'), but only for certain types of clinical questions (see Box 3.2 and sections 'Cohort studies', 'Case-control studies', 'Cross-sectional surveys' and 'Case reports'). The questions that best lend themselves to the RCT design all relate to *interventions*, and are mainly concerned with therapy or prevention. It should be

---

Box 3.3 Advantages of the randomised controlled trial design

1. Allows rigorous evaluation of a single variable (e.g. effect of drug treatment versus placebo) in a precisely defined patient group (e.g. post-menopausal women aged 50–60 years).
2. Prospective design (i.e. data are collected on events which happen *after* you decide to do the study).
3. Uses hypotheticodeductive reasoning (i.e. seeks to falsify, rather than confirm, its own hypothesis; see section 'Three preliminary questions to get your bearings').
4. Potentially eradicates bias by comparing two otherwise identical groups (but see subsequent text and section 'Was systematic bias avoided or minimised?').
5. Allows for meta-analysis (combining the numerical results of several similar trials) at a later date; see section 'Ten questions to ask about a paper that claims to validate a diagnostic or screening test').

Box 3.4 Disadvantages of the randomised controlled trial design

Expensive and time-consuming, hence, in practice,

- many RCTs are either never carried out, are performed on too few patients or are undertaken for too short a period (see section 'Were preliminary statistical questions addressed?');
- most RCTs are funded by large research bodies (university or government-sponsored) or drug companies, who ultimately dictate the research agenda;
- surrogate endpoints may not reflect outcomes that are important to patients (see section 'Surrogate endpoints').

May introduce 'hidden bias', especially through

- imperfect randomisation (see preceding text);
- failure to randomise all eligible patients (clinician only offers participation in the trial to patients she/he considers will respond well to the intervention);
- failure to blind assessors to randomisation status of patients (see section 'Was assessment 'blind'?').

remembered, however, that even when we are looking at therapeutic interventions, and especially when we are not, there are a number of important disadvantages associated with randomised trials (see Box 3.4) [11, 12].

Remember, too, that the results of an RCT may have limited applicability as a result of exclusion criteria (rules about who may not be entered into the study), inclusion bias (selection of trial participants from a group that is unrepresentative of everyone with the condition (see section 'Whom is the study about?')), refusal (or inability) of certain patient groups to give consent to be included in the trial, analysis of only pre-defined 'objective' endpoints which may exclude important qualitative aspects of the intervention (see Chapter 12) and publication bias (i.e. the selective publication of positive results, often but not always because the organisation that funded the research stands to gain or lose depending on the findings [9, 10]). Furthermore, RCTs can be well or badly managed [2], and, once published, their results are open to distortion by an over-enthusiastic scientific community or by a public eager for a new wonder drug [13]. While all these problems might also occur with other trial designs, they may be particularly pertinent when an RCT is being sold to you as, methodologically speaking, whiter than white.

There are, in addition, many situations in which RCTs are unnecessary, impractical or inappropriate:

RCTs are unnecessary
- when a clearly successful intervention for an otherwise fatal condition is discovered;
- when a previous RCT or meta-analysis has given a definitive result (either positive or negative – see section 'Probability and confidence'). Arguably, it is actually *unethical* to ask patients to be randomised to a clinical trial without first conducting a systematic literature review to see whether the trial needs to be carried out at all.

RCTs are impractical
- where it would be unethical to seek consent to randomise (see section 'A note on ethical considerations');
- where the number of participants needed to demonstrate a significant difference between the groups is prohibitively high (see section 'Were preliminary statistical questions addressed?');

RCTs are inappropriate
- where the study is looking at the prognosis of a disease. For this analysis, the appropriate route to best evidence is a longitudinal survey of a properly assembled *inception cohort* (see section 'Cross-sectional surveys');
- where the study is looking at the validity of a diagnostic or screening test. For this analysis, the appropriate route to best evidence is a *cross-sectional survey* of patients clinically suspected of harbouring the relevant disorder (see section 'Cross-sectional surveys' and Chapter 7);
- where the study is looking at a 'quality of care' issue in which the criteria for 'success' have not yet been established. For example, an RCT comparing medical versus surgical methods of abortion might assess 'success' in terms of number of patients achieving complete evacuation, amount of bleeding and pain level. The patients, however, might decide that other aspects of the procedure are important, such as knowing in advance how long the procedure will take, not seeing or feeling the abortus come out, and so on. For this analysis, the appropriate route to best evidence is *qualitative research methods* (see Chapter 12).

All these issues have been discussed in great depth by clinical epidemiologists, who remind us that to turn our noses up at the non-randomised trial may indicate scientific naiveté and not, as many people routinely assume, intellectual rigour [11]. You might also like to look up the emerging science of *pragmatic* RCTs – a methodology for taking account of practical, real-world challenges so that the findings of your trial will be more relevant to that real world when the trial is finished [14]. See also section 'What information to expect in a paper describing a randomised controlled trial: the CONSORT statement' where I introduce the Consolidated Standards of Reporting Trials (CONSORT) statement for presenting the findings of RCTs.

Cohort studies

In a cohort study, two (or more) groups of people are selected on the basis of differences in their exposure to a particular agent (such as a vaccine, a surgical procedure or an environmental toxin), and followed up to see how many in each group develop a particular disease, complication or other outcome. The follow-up period in cohort studies is generally measured in years (and some-times in decades) because that is how long many diseases, especially cancer, take to develop. Note that RCTs are usually begun on people who already have a disease, whereas most cohort studies are begun on people who may or may not develop disease.

A special type of cohort study may also be used to determine the prognosis of a disease (i.e. what is likely to happen to someone who has it). A group of people who have all been diagnosed as having an early stage of the disease or a positive screening test (see Chapter 7) is assembled (the inception cohort) and followed up on repeated occasions to see the incidence (new cases per year) and time course of different outcomes. (Here is a definition that you should commit to memory if you can: *incidence* is the number of new cases of a dis-ease per year, whereas *prevalence* is the overall proportion of the population who suffer from the disease.)

The world's most famous cohort study, whose authors all won knighthoods, was undertaken by Sir Austen Bradford Hill, Sir Richard Doll and, latterly, Sir Richard Peto. They followed up 40 000 male British doctors divided into four cohorts (non-smokers, and light, moderate and heavy smokers) using both all-cause (any death) and cause-specific (death from a particular dis-ease) mortality as outcome measures. Publication of their 10-year interim results in 1964 [15], which showed a substantial excess in both lung cancer mortality and all-cause mortality in smokers, with a 'dose–response' rela-tionship (i.e. the more you smoke, the worse your chances of getting lung cancer), went a long way to demonstrating that the link between smoking and ill health was causal rather than coincidental. The 20-year [16], 40-year [17] and 50-year [18] results of this momentous study (which achieved an impressive 94% follow-up of those recruited in 1951 and not known to have died) illustrate both the perils of smoking and the strength of evidence that can be obtained from a properly conducted cohort study.

Given here are clinical questions that should be addressed by a cohort study.

- Does smoking cause lung cancer?
- Does the contraceptive pill 'cause' breast cancer? (Note, once again, that the word 'cause' is a loaded and potentially misleading term. As Guillebaud has argued in his excellent book 'The Pill … '[19], if a thousand women went on the oral contraceptive pill tomorrow, some of them would get breast cancer. But some of those would have got it anyway. The question that epidemiologists try to answer through cohort studies is, 'what is the *additional* risk of developing breast cancer which this woman would run by taking the pill, over and above the baseline risk attributable to her own hormonal balance, family history, diet, alcohol intake, and so on?'.)
- Does high blood pressure get better over time?
- What happens to infants who have been born very prematurely, in terms of subsequent physical development and educational achievement?

Case–control studies

In a case–control study, patients with a particular disease or condition are identified and 'matched' with controls (patients with some other disease, the general population, neighbours or relatives). Data are then collected (e.g. by searching back through these people's medical records, or by asking them to recall their own history) on past exposure to a possible causal agent for the disease. Like cohort studies, case–control studies are generally concerned with the aetiology of a disease (i.e. what causes it), rather than its treatment. They lie lower down the conventional hierarchy of evidence (see subsequent text), but this design is usually the only option when studying rare conditions. An important source of difficulty (and potential bias) in a case–control study is the precise definition of who counts as a 'case', because one misallocated individual may substantially influence the results (see section 'Was systematic bias avoided or minimised?'). In addition, such a design cannot demonstrate causality – in other words, the *association* of A with B in a case–control study does not prove that A has *caused* B.

Clinical questions that should be addressed by a case–control study are listed here.

- Does the prone sleeping position increase the risk of cot death (sudden infant death syndrome)?
- Does whooping cough vaccine cause brain damage? (see section 'Was systematic bias avoided or minimised?').
- Do overhead power cables cause leukaemia?

Cross-sectional surveys

We have probably all been asked to take part in a survey, even if it was only a woman in the street asking us which brand of toothpaste we prefer. Surveys conducted by epidemiologists are run along essentially the same lines: a representative sample of participants is recruited and then interviewed, examined or otherwise studied to gain answers to a specific clinical (or other) question. In cross-sectional surveys, data are collected at a single time point but may refer retrospectively to health experiences in the past – for example, the study of patients' medical records to see how often their blood pressure has been recorded in the past 5 years.

A cross-sectional survey should address the following clinical questions .
• What is the 'normal' height of a 3-year-old child? This, like other questions about the range of normality, can be answered simply by measuring the height of enough healthy 3-year-olds. But such an exercise does not answer the related clinical question 'when should an unusually short child be investigated for disease?' because, as in almost all biological measurements, the physiological (normal) overlaps with the pathological (abnormal). This problem is discussed further in section 'Likelihood ratios'.
• What do psychiatric nurses believe about the value of antidepressant drugs and talking therapies in the treatment of severe depression?
• Is it true that 'half of all cases of diabetes are undiagnosed'? This an example of the more general question, 'What is the prevalence (proportion of people with the condition) of this disease in this community?' The only way of finding the answer is to do the definitive diagnostic test on a representative sample of the population.

Case reports

A case report describes the medical history of a single patient in the form of a story ('Mrs B is a 54 year old secretary who developed chest pain in June 2010 … '). Case reports are often run together to form a *case series*, in which the medical histories of more than one patient with a particular condition are described to illustrate an aspect of the condition, the treatment or, most commonly these days, adverse reaction to treatment.

Although this type of research is traditionally considered to be relatively weak as scientific evidence (see section 'The traditional hierarchy of evidence'), a great deal of information that would be lost in a clinical trial or survey can be conveyed in a case report (see Chapter 12). In addition, case reports are immediately understandable by non-academic clinicians and by the lay public. They can, if necessary, be written up and published within days, which gives them a definite edge over clinical trials (whose gestation period can run into years) or meta-analyses (even longer). There are certainly good theoretical grounds for the reinstatement of the humble case report as a useful and valid contribution to medical science, not least because the story is one of the best vehicles for *making sense* of a complex clinical situation. Richard Smith, who edited the British Medical Journal for 20 years, recently set up a new journal called *Cases* dedicated entirely to 'anecdotal' accounts of single clinical cases (see http://casesjournal.com/casesjournal).

The following are clinical situations in which a case report or case series is an appropriate type of study.

• A doctor notices that two babies born in his hospital have absent limbs (phocomelia). Both mothers had taken a new drug (thalidomide) in early pregnancy. The doctor wishes to alert his colleagues worldwide to the possibility of drug-related damage as quickly as possible [20]. (Anyone who thinks 'quick and dirty' case reports are never scientifically justified should remember this example.)

• A previously healthy patient develops spontaneous bacterial peritonitis – an unusual problem that the average doctor might see once in 10 years. The clinical team looking after her search the literature for research evidence and develop what they believe is an evidence-based management plan. The patient recovers well. The team decide to write this story up as a lesson for other clinicians – a so-called evidence-based case report [21].

The traditional hierarchy of evidence

Standard notation for the relative weight carried by the different types of primary study when making decisions about clinical interventions (the 'hierarchy of evidence') puts them in the given order.

1. Systematic reviews and meta-analyses (see Chapter 9);
2. RCTs with definitive results (i.e. confidence intervals that do not overlap the threshold clinically significant effect (see section 'Probability and confidence'));
3. RCTs with non-definitive results [i.e. a point estimate that suggests a clinically significant effect but with confidence intervals overlapping the threshold for this effect (see section 'Probability and confidence')];
4. Cohort studies;
5. Case–control studies;
6. Cross-sectional surveys;
7. Case reports.

The pinnacle of the hierarchy is, quite properly, reserved for secondary research papers, in which all the primary studies on a particular subject have been hunted out and critically appraised according to rigorous criteria (see Chapter 9). Note, however, that not even the most hard-line protagonist of EBM would place a sloppy meta-analysis or an RCT that was seriously methodologically flawed above a large, well-designed cohort study. And as Chapter 12 shows, many important and valid studies in the field of qualitative research do not feature in this particular hierarchy of evidence at all.

In other words, evaluating the potential contribution of a particular study to medical science requires considerably more effort than is needed to check off its basic design against the above-mentioned 7-point scale. A more recent publication on hierarchies of evidence suggests we should grade studies on four dimensions: risk of bias, consistency, directness and precision – an approach that would complicate any simple pyramid of evidence [22]. The take-home message is, don't apply the hierarchy of evidence mechanically – it's only a rule of thumb.

A more complex representation of the hierarchy of evidence geared to the domain of the question (therapy/prevention, diagnosis, harm, prognosis) was drawn up by a group of us in 2011 [23] and is available for download on the Centre for Evidence-Based Medicine website (http://www.cebm.net /index.aspx?o=5653). But before you look that one up, make sure you are clear on the traditional (basic) hierarchy described in this section.

A note on ethical considerations

When I was a junior doctor, I got a job in a world-renowned teaching hospital. One of my humble tasks was seeing the geriatric (elderly) patients in casualty. I was soon invited out to lunch by two charming mid-career doctors, who (I later realised) were seeking my help with their research. In return for getting my name on the paper, I was to take a rectal biopsy (i.e. cut out a small piece of tissue from the rectum) on any patient over the age of 90 who had consti-pation. I asked for a copy of the consent form that patients would be asked to sign. When they assured me that the average 90-year-old would hardly notice the procedure, I smelt a rat and refused to cooperate with their project.

At the time, I was naïvely unaware of the seriousness of the offence being planned by these doctors. Doing *any* research, particularly that which involves invasive procedures, on vulnerable and sick patients without full consideration of ethical issues is both a criminal offence and potential grounds for a doctor to be 'struck off' the medical register. Getting formal ethical approval for one's research study (for UK readers, see corec.org.uk), and ensuring that the research is properly run and adequately monitored (a set of tasks and responsibilities known as *research governance* [24–26]) can be an enormous bureaucratic hurdle. Ethical issues were, sadly, sometimes ignored in the past in research in babies, the elderly, those with learning difficulties and those unable to protest (e.g. prisoners and the military), leading to some infamous research scandals [24].

These days, most editors routinely refuse to publish research that has not been approved by a research ethics committee. Note, however, that heavy-handed approaches to research governance by official bodies may be ethically questionable. Neurologist and researcher Professor Charles Warlow [27] argued some years ago that the overemphasis on 'informed consent' by well-intentioned research ethics committees has been the kiss of death to research into head injuries, strokes and other acute brain problems (in which, clearly, the person is in no position to consider the personal pros and cons of taking part in a research study). More recently, exasperated researchers published a salutary tale entitled 'Bureaucracy stifles medical research in Britain' [28]. The bottom line message for this book is: make sure that the study you are reading about has had ethical approval, while also sympathising with researchers who have had to 'jump through hoops' to get it.

References

1 Altman DG. The scandal of poor medical research. BMJ: British Medical Journal 1994;**308**(6924):283.

2 Altman DG. Poor-quality medical research. JAMA: The Journal of the American Medical Association 2002;**287**(21):2765–7.

3 Godlee F, Jefferson T, Callaham M, et al. *Peer review in health sciences*. London: BMJ Books, 2003.

4 Popper KR. *The logic of scientific discovery*. Abingdon, UK: Psychology Press, 2002.

5 Anon. Randomised trial of intravenous streptokinase, aspirin, both, or neither among 17187 cases of suspected acute myocardial infarction: ISIS-2. (ISIS-2 Collaborative Group). Lancet 1988;**ii**:349–60.

6 Lee A, Joynt GM, Ho AM, et al. Tips for teachers of evidence-based medicine: making sense of decision analysis using a decision tree. Journal of General Internal Medicine 2009;**24**(5):642–8.

7 Drummond MF, Sculpher MJ, Torrance GW. *Methods for the economic evaluation of health care programs*. Oxford: Oxford University Press, 2005.

8 Fletcher W. Rice and beriberi: preliminary report of an experiment conducted at the Kuala Lumpur Lunatic Asylum. Lancet 1907;**1**:1776.

9 Sterne JA, Egger M, Smith GD. Systematic reviews in health care: investigating and dealing with publication and other biases in meta-analysis. BMJ: British Medical Journal 2001;**323**(7304):101.

10 Cuff A. Sources of Bias in Clinical Trials. 2013. http://applyingcriticality.wordpress .com/2013/06/19/sources-of-bias-in-clinical-trials/ (accessed 26th June 2013).

11 Kaptchuk TJ. The double-blind, randomized, placebo-controlled trial: gold standard or golden calf? Journal of Clinical Epidemiology 2001;**54**(6):541–9.

12 Berwick D. Broadening the view of evidence-based medicine. Quality and Safety in Health Care 2005;**14**(5):315–6.

13 McCormack J, Greenhalgh T. Seeing what you want to see in randomised controlled trials: versions and perversions of UKPDS data. United Kingdom prospective diabetes study. BMJ: British Medical Journal 2000;**320**(7251):1720–3.

14 Eldridge S. Pragmatic trials in primary health care: what, when and how? Family Practice 2010;**27**(6):591–2 doi: 10.1093/fampra/cmq099.

15 Doll R, Hill AB. Mortality in relation to smoking: ten years' observations of British doctors. BMJ: British Medical Journal 1964;**1**(5395):1399.

16 Doll R, Peto R. Mortality in relation to smoking: 20 years' observations on male British doctors. BMJ: British Medical Journal 1976;**2**(6051):1525.

17 Doll R, Peto R, Wheatley K, et al. Mortality in relation to smoking: 40 years' observations on male British doctors. BMJ: British Medical Journal 1994;**309**(6959):901–11.

18 Doll R, Peto R, Boreham J, et al. Mortality in relation to smoking: 50 years' observations on male British doctors. BMJ: British Medical Journal 2004;**328**(7455):1519.

19 Guillebaud J, MacGregor A. *The pill and other forms of hormonal contraception.* USA: Oxford University Press, 2009.

20 McBride WG. Thalidomide and congenital abnormalities. Lancet 1961;**2**:1358.

21 Soares-Weiser K, Paul M, Brezis M, et al. Evidence based case report. Antibiotic treatment for spontaneous bacterial peritonitis. BMJ: British Medical Journal 2002;**324**(7329):100–2.

22 Owens DK, Lohr KN, Atkins D, et al. AHRQ series paper 5: grading the strength of a body of evidence when comparing medical interventions – agency for healthcare research and quality and the effective health-care program. Journal of Clinical Epidemiology 2010;**63**(5):513–23 doi: 10.1016/j.jclinepi.2009.03.009.

23 Howick J, Chalmers I, Glasziou P, et al. *The 2011 Oxford CEBM levels of evidence (introductory document).* Oxford: Oxford Centre for Evidence-Based Medicine, 2011.

24 Slowther A, Boynton P, Shaw S. Research governance: ethical issues. JRSM: Journal of the Royal Society of Medicine 2006;**99**(2):65–72.

25 Shaw S, Boynton PM, Greenhalgh T. Research governance: where did it come from, what does it mean? JRSM: Journal of the Royal Society of Medicine 2005;**98**(11):496–502.

26 Shaw S, Barrett G. Research governance: regulating risk and reducing harm? JRSM: Journal of the Royal Society of Medicine 2006;**99**(1):14–9.

27 Warlow C. Over-regulation of clinical research: a threat to public health. Clinical Medicine 2005;**5**(1):33–8.

28 Snooks H, Hutchings H, Seagrove A, et al. Bureaucracy stifles medical research in Britain: a tale of three trials. BMC Medical Research Methodology 2012;**12**(1):122.

Chapter 4 **Assessing methodological quality**

As I argued in section 'The science of "trashing" papers', a paper will sink or swim on the strength of its methods section. This chapter considers five essential questions which should form the basis of your decision to 'bin' it outright (because of fatal methodological flaws), interpret its findings cautiously (because the methods were less than robust) or trust it completely (because you can't fault the methods at all). These five questions – was the study original, whom is it about, was it well designed, was systematic bias avoided (i.e. was the study adequately 'controlled') and was it large enough and continued for long enough to make the results credible – are considered in turn.

Was the study original?

There is, in theory, no point in testing a scientific hypothesis that someone else has already proved one way or the other. But in real life, science is seldom so cut and dried. Only a tiny proportion of medical research breaks entirely new ground, and an equally tiny proportion repeats exactly the steps of previous workers. The majority of research studies will tell us (if they are methodologically sound) that a particular hypothesis is slightly more or less likely to be correct than it was before we added our piece to the wider jigsaw. Hence, it may be perfectly valid to do a study that is, on the face of it, 'unoriginal'. Indeed, the whole science of meta-analysis depends on there being more than one study in the literature that have addressed the same question in pretty much the same way.

The practical question to ask, then, about a new piece of research, is not 'has anyone ever conducted a similar study before?', but 'does this new research add to the literature in any way?' A list of such examples is given here.

How to Read a Paper: The Basics of Evidence-Based Medicine, Fifth Edition. Trisha Greenhalgh.
© 2014 John Wiley & Sons, Ltd. Published 2014 by John Wiley & Sons, Ltd.

- Is this study bigger, continued for longer, or otherwise more substantial than the previous one(s)?
- Are the methods of this study any more rigorous (in particular, does it address any specific methodological criticisms of previous studies)?
- Will the numerical results of this study add significantly to a meta-analysis of previous studies?
- Is the population studied different in any way (e.g. has the study looked at different ethnic groups, ages or gender than have previous studies)?
- Is the clinical issue addressed of sufficient importance, and does there exist sufficient doubt in the minds of the public or key decision-makers, to make new evidence 'politically' desirable even when it is not strictly scientifically necessary?

Whom is the study about?

One of the first papers that ever caught my eye was entitled 'But will it help *my* patients with myocardial infarction?' [1]. I don't remember the details of the article, but it opened my eyes to the fact that research on someone else's patients may not have a take-home message for my own practice. This is not mere xenophobia. The main reasons why the participants (Sir Iain Chalmers has argued forcefully against calling them 'patients') [2] in a clinical trial or survey might differ from patients in 'real life' are listed here.

(a) They were more, or less, ill than the patients you see.

(b) They were from a different ethnic group, or lived a different lifestyle, from your own patients.

(c) They received more (or different) attention during the study than you could ever hope to give your patients.

(d) Unlike most real-life patients, they had nothing wrong with them apart from the condition being studied.

(e) None of them smoked, drank alcohol or were taking the contraceptive pill.

Hence, before swallowing the results of any paper whole, here are some questions that you should ask yourself.

1. *How were the participants recruited?* If you wanted to do a questionnaire survey of the views of users of the hospital casualty department, you could recruit respondents by putting an ad in the local newspaper. However, this method would be a good example of *recruitment bias* because the sample you obtain would be skewed in favour of users who were highly motivated to answer your questions and liked to read newspapers. You would do better to issue a questionnaire to every user (or to a one in ten sample of users) who turned up on a particular day.

2. *Who was included in the study?* In the past, clinical trials routinely excluded people with coexisting illness, those who did not speak English, those taking certain other medication and people who could not read the consent form. This approach may be experimentally clean but because clinical trial results will be used to guide practice in relation to wider patient groups, it is actually scientifically flawed. The results of pharmacokinetic studies of new drugs in 23-year-old healthy male volunteers will clearly not be applicable to the average elderly female! This issue, which has been a bugbear of some doctors and scientists for decades, has more recently been taken up by the patients themselves, most notably in the plea from patient support groups for a broadening of inclusion criteria in trials of anti-AIDS drugs [3].

3. *Who was excluded from the study?* For example, an randomised controlled trial may be restricted to patients with moderate or severe forms of a disease such as heart failure – a policy that could lead to false conclusions about the treatment of *mild* heart failure. This has important practical implications when clinical trials performed on hospital outpatients are used to dictate 'best practice' in primary care, where the spectrum of disease is generally milder.

4. *Were the participants studied in 'real-life' circumstances?* For example, were they admitted to hospital purely for observation? Did they receive lengthy and detailed explanations of the potential benefits of the intervention? Were they given the telephone number of a key research worker? Did the company who funded the research provide new equipment that would not be available to the ordinary clinician? These factors would not invalidate the study, but they may cast doubts on the applicability of its findings to your own practice.

Was the design of the study sensible?

Although the terminology of research trial design can be forbidding, much of what is grandly termed *critical appraisal* is plain common sense. Personally, I assess the basic design of a clinical trial via two questions.

What specific intervention or other manoeuvre was being considered, and what was it being compared with? This is one of the most fundamental questions in appraising any paper. It is tempting to take published statements at face value, but remember that authors frequently misrepresent (usually subconsciously rather than deliberately) what they actually did, and overestimate its originality and potential importance. In the examples in Table 4.1, I have used hypothetical statements so as not to cause offence, but they are all based on similar mistakes seen in print.

Table 4.1 Examples of problematic descriptions in the methods section of a paper

What the authors said	What they should have said (or should have done)	An example of
'We measured how often GPs ask patients whether they smoke.'	'We looked in patients' medical records and counted how many had had their smoking status recorded.'	Assumption that medical records are 100% accurate.
'We measured how doctors treat low back pain.'	'We measured what doctors say they do when faced with a patient with low back pain.'	Assumption that what doctors say they do reflects what they actually do.
'We compared a nicotine-replacement patch with placebo.'	'Participants in the intervention group were asked to apply a patch containing 15 mg nicotine twice daily; those in the control group received identical-looking patches.'	Failure to state dose of drug or nature of placebo.
'We asked 100 teenagers to participate in our survey of sexual attitudes.'	'We approached 147 white American teenagers aged 12–18 (85 males) at a summer camp; 100 of them (31 males) agreed to participate.'	Failure to give sufficient information about participants. (Note in this example the figures indicate a recruitment bias towards women.)
'We randomised patients to either "individual care plan" or "usual care."'	'The intervention group were offered an individual care plan consisting of ....; control patients were offered ....'	Failure to give sufficient information about intervention. (Enough information should be given to allow the study to be repeated by other workers.)
'To assess the value of an educational leaflet, we gave the intervention group a leaflet and a telephone helpline number. Controls received neither.'	If the study is purely to assess the value of the leaflet, both groups should have got the helpline number.	Failure to treat groups equally apart from the specific intervention.
'We measured the use of vitamin C in the prevention of the common cold.'	A systematic literature search would have found numerous previous studies on this subject (see When is a review systematic? section).	Unoriginal study.

What outcome was measured, and how? If you had an incurable disease, for which a pharmaceutical company claimed to have produced a new wonder drug, you would measure the efficacy of the drug in terms of whether it made you live longer (and, perhaps, whether life was *worth* living given your condition and any side effects of the medication). You would not be too interested in the levels of some obscure enzyme in your blood that the manufacturer assured you were a reliable indicator of your chances of survival. The use of such *surrogate endpoints* is discussed further in the section 'Surrogate endpoints' on page 81.

The measurement of symptomatic (e.g. pain), functional (e.g. mobility), psychological (e.g. anxiety) or social (e.g. inconvenience) effects of an intervention is fraught with even more problems. The methodology of developing, administering and interpreting such 'soft' outcome measures is beyond the scope of this book. But, in general, you should always look for evidence in the paper that the outcome measure has been objectively validated – that is, that someone has demonstrated that the 'outcome measure' used in the study has been shown to measure what it purports to measure, and that changes in this outcome measure adequately reflect changes in the status of the patient. Remember that what is important in the eyes of the doctor may not be valued so highly by the patient, and vice versa. One of the most exciting developments in evidence based medicine (EBM) in recent years is the emerging science of patient-reported outcomes measures, which I cover in the section 'PROMs' on page 223.

Was systematic bias avoided or minimised?

Systematic bias is defined by epidemiologists as anything that erroneously influences the conclusions about groups and distorts comparisons [4]. Whether the design of a study is an randomised control trial (RCT), a non-randomised comparative trial, a cohort study or a case–control study, the aim should be for the groups being compared to be as like one another as possible except for the particular difference being examined. They should, as far as possible, receive the same explanations, have the same contacts with health professionals, and be assessed the same number of times by the same assessors, using the same outcome measures [5, 6]. Different study designs call for different steps to reduce systematic bias.

Randomised controlled trials

In an RCT, systematic bias is (in theory) avoided by selecting a sample of participants from a particular population and allocating them randomly to the different groups. Section 'Randomised controlled trials' describes some ways in which bias can creep into even this gold standard of clinical trial design, and Figure 4.1 summarises particular sources to check for.

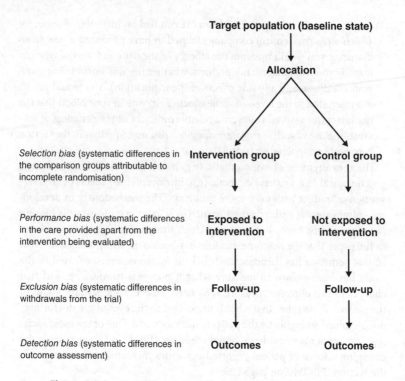

Figure 4.1 Sources of bias to check for in a randomised controlled trial.

Non-randomised controlled clinical trials

I once chaired a seminar in which a multidisciplinary group of students from the medical, nursing, pharmacy and allied professions were presenting the results of several in-house research studies. All but one of the studies presented were of comparative, but non-randomised, design – that is, one group of patients (say, hospital outpatients with asthma) had received one intervention (say, an educational leaflet), while another group (say, patients attending general practitioner (GP) surgeries with asthma) had received another intervention (say, group educational sessions). I was surprised how many of the presenters believed that their study was, or was equivalent to, an RCT. In other words, these commendably enthusiastic and committed young researchers were blind to the most obvious bias of all: they were comparing two groups that had inherent, self-selected differences even before the intervention was applied (as well as having all the additional potential sources of bias listed in Figure 4.1 for RCTs).

As a general rule, if the paper you are looking at is a non-randomised controlled clinical trial, you must use your common sense to decide if the baseline differences between the intervention and control groups are likely to have been so great as to invalidate any differences ascribed to the effects of the intervention. This is, in fact, almost always the case [7]. Sometimes, the authors of such a paper will list the important features of each group (such as mean age, sex ratio and markers of disease severity) in a table to allow you to compare these differences yourself.

Cohort studies

The selection of a comparable control group is one of the most difficult decisions facing the authors of an observational (cohort or case–control) study. Few, if any, cohort studies, for example, succeed in identifying two groups of subjects who are equal in age, gender mix, socioeconomic status, presence of coexisting illness and so on, with the single difference being their exposure to the agent being studied. In practice, much of the 'controlling' in cohort studies occurs at the analysis stage, where complex statistical adjustment is made for baseline differences in key variables. Unless this is performed adequately, statistical tests of probability and confidence intervals (see section 'Probability and confidence') will be dangerously misleading [6, 7].

This problem is illustrated by the various cohort studies on the risks and benefits of alcohol, which have consistently demonstrated a J-shaped relationship between alcohol intake and mortality. The best outcome (in terms of premature death) lies with the cohort group who are moderate drinkers [8]. Self-confessed teetotalers, it seems, are significantly more likely to die young than the average person who drinks three or four drinks a day.

But can we assume that teetotallers are, *on average*, identical to moderate drinkers except for the amount they drink? We certainly can't. As we all know, the teetotal population includes those who have been ordered to give up alcohol on health grounds ('sick quitters'), those who, for health or other reasons, have cut out a host of additional items from their diet and lifestyle, those from certain religious or ethnic groups which would be under-represented in the other cohorts (notably Muslims and Seventh Day Adventists), and those who drink like fish but choose to lie about it.

The details of how these different features of teetotalism were controlled for by the epidemiologists are discussed elsewhere [8, 9]. Interestingly, when I was writing the third edition of this book in 2005, the conclusion at that time was that even when due allowance was made in the analysis for potential confounding variables in people who described themselves as non-drinkers, these individuals' increased risk of premature mortality remained (i.e. the J curve was a genuine phenomenon) [8].

But by the time I wrote the fourth edition in 2010, a more sophisticated analysis of the various cohort studies (i.e. which controlled more carefully for 'sick quitters') had been published [9]. It showed that, all other things being equal, teetotallers are no more likely to contract heart disease than moderate drinkers (hence, the famous 'J curve' may have been an artefact all along). Subsequently, a new meta-analysis purported to show that the J curve was a genuine phenomenon and alcohol was indeed protective in small quantities [10] – but a year later a new analysis of the same primary studies came to the opposite conclusion, having placed more weight on so-called methodological flaws [11]. Depending on your perspective, this could be one to discuss with your EBM colleagues over a beer.

Case–control studies

In case–control studies (in which, as I explained in section 'Case reports', the experiences of individuals with and without a particular disease are analysed retrospectively to identify exposure to possible causes of that disease), the process most open to bias is not the assessment of outcome, but the diagnosis of 'caseness' and the decision as to *when* the individual became a case.

A good example of this occurred a few years ago when legal action was brought against the manufacturers of the whooping cough (pertussis) vaccine, which was alleged to have caused neurological damage in a number of infants [12]. In order to answer the question 'Did the vaccine cause brain damage?', a case–control study had been undertaken in which a 'case' was defined as an infant who, previously well, had exhibited fits or other signs suggestive of brain damage within 1 week of receiving the vaccine. A control was an infant of the same age and sex taken from the same immunisation register, who had received immunisation and who may or may not have developed symptoms at some stage.

New onset of features of brain damage in apparently normal babies is extremely rare, but it does happen, and the link with recent immunisation could conceivably be coincidental. Furthermore, heightened public anxiety about the issue could have biased the recall of parents and health professionals so that infants whose neurological symptoms predated, or occurred some time after, the administration of pertussis vaccine, might be wrongly classified as cases. The judge in the court case ruled that misclassification of three such infants as 'cases' rather than controls led to the overestimation of the harm attributable to whooping cough vaccine by a factor of three [12]. Although this ruling has subsequently been challenged, the principle stands – that assignment of 'caseness' in a case–control study must be performed rigorously and objectively if systematic bias is to be avoided.

Was assessment 'blind'?

Even the most rigorous attempt to achieve a comparable control group will be wasted effort if the people who assess outcome (e.g. those who judge whether someone is still clinically in heart failure, or who say whether an X-ray is 'improved' from last time) know which group the patient they are assessing was allocated to. If you believe that the evaluation of clinical signs and the interpretation of diagnostic tests such as ECGs and X-rays is 100% objective, you haven't been in the game very long [13].

The chapter 'The Clinical Examination' in Sackett and colleagues' book 'Clinical epidemiology: a basic science for clinical medicine' [14] provides substantial evidence that when examining patients, doctors find what they expect and hope to find. It is rare for two competent clinicians to reach complete agreement for any given aspect of the physical examination or interpretation of any diagnostic test. The level of agreement beyond chance between two observers can be expressed mathematically as the Kappa score, with a score of 1.0 indicating perfect agreement. Kappa scores for specialists in the field assessing the height of a patient's jugular venous pressure, classifying diabetic retinopathy from retinal photographs and interpreting a mammogram X-ray, were, respectively, 0.42, 0.55 and 0.67 [14].

This digression into clinical disagreement should have persuaded you that efforts to keep assessors 'blind' (or to avoid offence to the visually impaired, *masked*), to the group allocation of their patients are far from superfluous. If, for example, I knew that a patient had been randomised to an active drug to lower blood pressure rather than to a placebo, I might be more likely to re-check a reading that was surprisingly high. This is an example of *performance bias*, which, along with other pitfalls for the unblinded assessor, are listed in Figure 4.1.

An excellent example of controlling for bias by adequate 'blinding' was published in the *Lancet* a few years ago [15]. Majeed and colleagues performed an RCT that demonstrated, in contrast with the findings of several previous studies, that the recovery time (days in hospital, days off work and time to resume full activity) after laparoscopic removal of the gallbladder (the 'keyhole surgery' approach) was no quicker than that associated with the traditional open operation. The discrepancy between this trial and its predecessors may have been because of the authors' meticulous attempt to reduce bias (see Figure 4.1). The patients were not randomised until after induction of general anaesthesia. Neither the patients nor their carers were aware of which operation had been performed, as all patients left the operating theatre with identical dressings (complete with blood stains!). These findings challenge previous authors to ask themselves whether it was expectation bias (see section 'Ten questions to ask about a paper that claims to validate a diagnostic or screening test'), rather than swifter recovery, which spurred doctors to discharge the laparoscopic surgery group earlier.

Were preliminary statistical questions addressed?

As a non-statistician, I tend only to look for three numbers in the methods section of a paper.
(a) The size of the sample;
(b) The duration of follow-up; and
(c) The completeness of follow-up.

Sample size

One crucial prerequisite before embarking on a clinical trial is to perform a sample size ('power') calculation. A trial should be big enough to have a high chance of detecting, as statistically significant, a worthwhile effect if it exists, and thus to be reasonably sure that no benefit exists if it is not found in the trial.

In order to calculate sample size, the clinician must decide two things.

• The level of difference between the two groups that would constitute a *clinically significant* effect. Note that this may not be the same as a statistically significant effect. To cite an example from a famous clinical trial of hypertension therapy, you could administer a new drug that lowered blood pressure by around 10 mmHg, and the effect would be a statistically significant lowering of the chances of developing stroke (i.e. the odds are less than 1 in 20 that the reduced incidence occurred by chance) [16]. However, if the people being asked to take this drug had only mildly raised blood pressure and no other major risk factors for stroke (i.e. they were relatively young, not diabetic, had normal cholesterol levels, etc.), this level of difference would only prevent around one stroke in every 850 patients treated – a clinical difference in risk which many patients would classify as not worth the hassle of taking the tablets. This was shown over 20 years ago – and confirmed by numerous studies since (see a recent Cochrane review [17]). Yet far too many doctors still treat their patients according to the *statistical* significance of the findings of mega trials rather than the clinical significance for their patient; hence (some argue), we now have a near-epidemic of over-treated mild hypertension [18].

• The mean and the standard deviation (abbreviated SD; see 'a' of section 'Have the authors set the scene correctly?') of the principal outcome variable.

If the outcome in question is an event (such as hysterectomy) rather than a quantity (such as blood pressure), the items of data required are the proportion of people experiencing the event in the population, and an estimate of what might constitute a clinically significant change in that proportion.

Once these items of data have been ascertained, the minimum sample size can be easily computed using standard formulae, nomograms or tables, which may be obtained from published papers [19], textbooks [20], free access websites (try http://www.macorr.com/ss_calculator.htm) or commercial statistical software packages (see, for example, http://www.ncss.com/pass.html). Hence, the researchers can, *before the trial begins*, work out how large a sample they will need in order to have a moderate, high or very high chance of detecting a true difference between the groups. The likelihood of detecting a true difference is known as the *power* of the study. It is common for studies to stipulate a power of between 80% and 90%. Hence, when reading a paper about an RCT, you should look for a sentence that reads something like this (which is taken from Majeed and colleagues' cholecystectomy paper described earlier) [15].

> For a 90% chance of detecting a difference of one night's stay in hospital using the Mann–Whitney U-test [see Chapter 5, Table 5.1], 100 patients were needed in each group (assuming SD of 2 nights). This gives a power greater than 90% for detecting a difference in operating times of 15 minutes, assuming a SD of 20 minutes.

If the paper you are reading does not give a sample size calculation *and* it appears to show that there is no difference between the intervention and control arms of the trial, you should extract from the paper (or directly from the authors) the information in (a) and (b) earlier and do the calculation yourself. Underpowered studies are ubiquitous in the medical literature, usually because the authors found it harder than they anticipated to recruit their participants. Such studies typically lead to a Type II or β error – that is, the erroneous conclusion that an intervention has no effect. (In contrast, the rarer Type I or α error is the conclusion that a difference is significant when, in fact, it is because of sampling error.)

Duration of follow-up

Even if the sample size itself was adequate, a study must be continued for long enough for the effect of the intervention to be reflected in the outcome variable. If the authors were looking at the effect of a new painkiller on the degree of post-operative pain, their study may only have needed a follow-up period of 48 h. On the other hand, if they were looking at the effect of nutritional supplementation in the preschool years on final adult height, follow-up should have been measured in decades.

Even if the intervention has demonstrated a significant difference between the groups after, say, 6 months, that difference may not be sustained. As many dieters know from bitter experience, strategies to reduce obesity often show dramatic results after 2 or 3 weeks, but if follow-up is continued for a year or more, the unfortunate participants have (more often than not) put most of the weight back on.

Completeness of follow-up

It has been shown repeatedly that participants who withdraw from research studies are less likely to have taken their tablets as directed, more likely to have missed their interim check-ups and more likely to have experienced side effects on any medication, than those who do not withdraw (incidentally, don't use the term *drop out* as this is pejorative). People who fail to complete questionnaires may feel differently about the issue (and probably less strongly) than those who send them back by return of post. People on a weight-reducing programme are more likely to continue coming back if they are actually losing weight.

The following are among the reasons patients withdraw (or are withdrawn by the researchers) from clinical trials.

1. Incorrect entry of patient into trial (i.e. researcher discovers during the trial that the patient should not have been randomised in the first place because he or she did not fulfil the entry criteria).
2. Suspected adverse reaction to the trial drug. Note that you should never look at the 'adverse reaction' rate in the intervention group without comparing it with that on placebo. Inert tablets bring people out in a rash surprisingly frequently.
3. Loss of participant motivation ('I don't want to take these tablets any more').
4. Clinical reasons (e.g. concurrent illness, pregnancy).
5. Loss to follow-up (e.g. participant moves away).
6. Death. Clearly, people who die will not attend for their outpatient appointments, so unless specifically accounted for they might be misclassified as withdrawals. This is one reason why studies with a low follow-up rate (say, below 70%) are generally considered untrustworthy.

Ignoring everyone who has failed to complete a clinical trial will bias the results, usually in favour of the intervention. It is, therefore, standard practice to analyse the results of comparative studies on an *intent-to-treat* basis. This means that all data on participants originally allocated to the intervention arm of the study, including those who withdrew before the trial finished, those who did not take their tablets and even those who subsequently received the control intervention for whatever reason, should be analysed along with data on the patients who followed the protocol throughout. Conversely, withdrawals from the placebo arm of the study should be analysed with those who faithfully took their placebo. If you look hard enough in a paper, you will usually find the sentence, 'results were analysed on an intent-to-treat basis', but you should not be reassured until you have checked and confirmed the figures yourself.

There are, in fact, a few situations when intent-to-treat analysis is, rightly, not used. The most common is the *efficacy* (*or per-protocol*) *analysis*, which is to explain the effects of the intervention itself, and is therefore of the treatment actually received. But even if the participants in an efficacy analysis are part of an RCT, for the purposes of the analysis they effectively constitute a cohort study (see section 'Cohort studies').

Summing up

Having worked through the Methods section of a paper, you should be able to tell yourself in a short paragraph what sort of study was performed, on how many participants, where the participants came from, what treatment or other intervention was offered, how long the follow-up period was (or, if a survey, what the response rate was) and what outcome measure(s) were used. You should also, at this stage, identify what statistical tests, if any, were used to analyse the data (see Chapter 5). If you are clear about these things before reading the rest of the paper, you will find the results easier to understand, interpret and, if appropriate, reject. You should be able to come up with descriptions such as those given here.

This paper describes an unblinded randomised trial, concerned with therapy, in 267 hospital outpatients aged between 58 and 93 years, in which four-layer compression bandaging was compared with standard single-layer dressings in the management of uncomplicated venous leg ulcers. Follow-up was six months. Percentage healing of the ulcer was measured from baseline in terms of the surface area of a tracing of the wound taken by the district nurse and calculated by a computer scanning device. Results were analysed using the Wilcoxon matched-pairs test.

This is a questionnaire survey of 963 general practitioners randomly selected from throughout the UK, in which they were asked their year of

*graduation from medical school and the level at which they would begin
treatment for essential hypertension. Response options on the structured
questionnaire were 'below 89 mm Hg', '90-99 mm Hg' and '100 mm Hg
or greater'.*

*Results were analysed using a Chi-squared test on a 3 × 2 table to see
whether the threshold for treating hypertension was related to whether
the doctor graduated from medical school before or after 1985.*

*This is a case report of a single patient with a suspected fatal adverse
drug reaction to the newly-released hypnotic drug Sleepol.*

When you have had a little practice in looking at the Methods section
of research papers along the lines suggested in this chapter, you will find
that it is only a short step to start using the checklists in Appendix 1, or the
more comprehensive Users' Guides to the Medical Literature (http://www
.cche.net/usersguides/main.asp). I will return to many of the issues discussed
here in Chapter 6, in relation to evaluating papers on trials of drug therapy
and other simple interventions.

References

1 Mitchell J. "But will it help my patients with myocardial infarction?" The implications of recent trials for everyday country folk British Medical Journal (Clinical
 Research Edition) 1982;**285**(6349):1140.
2 McCormack J, Greenhalgh T. Seeing what you want to see in randomised controlled trials: versions and perversions of UKPDS data. United Kingdom prospective diabetes study. BMJ: British Medical Journal 2000;**320**(7251):1720–3.
3 Phillips AN, Smith GD, Johnson MA. Will we ever know when to treat HIV infection? BMJ: British Medical Journal 1996;**313**(7057):608.
4 Coggon D, Barker D, Rose G. *Epidemiology for the uninitiated.* London: BMJ
 Books, 2009.
5 Cuff A. Sources of Bias in Clinical Trials. 2013. http://applyingcriticality.wordpress
 .com/2013/06/19/sources-of-bias-in-clinical-trials/ (accessed 26th June 2013).
6 Delgado-Rodríguez M, Llorca J. Bias. Journal of Epidemiology and Community
 Health 2004;**58**(8):635–41 doi: 10.1136/jech.2003.008466.
7 Britton A, McKee M, Black N, et al. Choosing between randomised and
 non-randomised studies: a systematic review. Health Technology Assessment
 (Winchester, England) 1998;**2**(13):i.
8 Rimm EB, Williams P, Fosher K, et al. Moderate alcohol intake and lower risk of
 coronary heart disease: meta-analysis of effects on lipids and haemostatic factors.
 BMJ: British Medical Journal 1999;**319**(7224):1523.

9 Fillmore KM, Stockwell T, Chikritzhs T, et al. Moderate alcohol use and reduced mortality risk: systematic error in prospective studies and new hypotheses. Annals of Epidemiology 2007;**17**(5):S16–23.

10 Ronksley PE, Brien SE, Turner BJ, et al. Association of alcohol consumption with selected cardiovascular disease outcomes: a systematic review and meta-analysis. BMJ: British Medical Journal 2011;**342**:d671.

11 Stockwell T, Greer A, Fillmore K, et al. How good is the science? BMJ: British Medical Journal 2012;**344**:e2276.

12 Bowie C. Lessons from the pertussis vaccine court trial. Lancet 1990;**335**(8686), 397–399.

13 Gawande A. *Complications: a surgeon's notes on an imperfect science*. London: Profile Books, 2010.

14 Sackett DL, Haynes RB, Tugwell P. *Clinical epidemiology: a basic science for clinical medicine*. Boston, USA: Little, Brown and Company, 1985.

15 Majeed A, Troy G, Smythe A, et al. Randomised, prospective, single-blind comparison of laparoscopic versus small-incision cholecystectomy. The Lancet 1996;**347**(9007):989–94.

16 MRC Working Party. Medical Research Council trial of treatment of hypertension in older adults: principal results. BMJ: British Medical Journal 1992;**304**:405–12.

17 Diao D, Wright JM, Cundiff DK, et al. Pharmacotherapy for mild hypertension. Cochrane Database of Systematic Reviews (Online) 2012;**8**:CD006742 doi: 10.1002/14651858.CD006742.pub2.

18 Spence D. Why do we overtreat hypertension? BMJ: British Medical Journal 2012;**345**:e5923 doi: 10.1136/bmj.e5923.

19 Charles P, Giraudeau B, Dechartres A, et al. Reporting of sample size calculation in randomised controlled trials: review. BMJ: British Medical Journal 2009;**338**:b1732.

20 Machin D, Campbell MJ, Tan S-B, et al. *Sample size tables for clinical studies*. Oxford: Wiley-Blackwell, 2011.

Chapter 5 **Statistics for the non-statistician**

How can non-statisticians evaluate statistical tests?

In this age where medicine leans increasingly on mathematics, no clinician can afford to leave the statistical aspects of a paper entirely to the 'experts'. If, like me, you believe yourself to be innumerate, remember that you do not need to be able to build a car in order to drive one. What you do need to know about statistical tests is which is the best test to use for common types of statistical questions. You need to be able to describe *in words* what the test does and in what circumstances it becomes invalid or inappropriate. Box 5.1 shows some frequently used 'tricks of the trade', which all of us need to be alert to (in our own as well as other people's practice).

The summary checklist in Appendix 1, explained in detail in the subsequent sections, constitute my own method for assessing the adequacy of a statistical analysis, which some readers will find too simplistic. If you do, please skip this section and turn either to a more comprehensive presentation for the non-statistician: the 'Basic Statistics for Clinicians' series in the *Canadian Medical Association Journal* [1–4], or to a more mainstream statistical textbook. When I asked my Twitter followers which statistics textbook they preferred, the post popular ones were these [5–7]. If you find statistics impossibly difficult, take these points one at a time and return to read the next point only when you feel comfortable with the previous ones. None of the points presupposes a detailed knowledge of the actual calculations involved.

The first question to ask, by the way, is, 'Have the authors used any statistical tests at all?' If they are presenting numbers and claiming that these numbers mean something, without using statistical methods to prove it, they are almost certainly skating on thin ice.

How to Read a Paper: The Basics of Evidence-Based Medicine, Fifth Edition. Trisha Greenhalgh.
© 2014 John Wiley & Sons, Ltd. Published 2014 by John Wiley & Sons, Ltd.

Box 5.1 Ten ways to cheat on statistical tests when writing up results

1. Throw all your data into a computer and report as significant any relationship where '$p < 0.05$' (see section 'Have "p-values" been calculated and interpreted appropriately?').
2. If baseline differences between the groups favour the intervention group, remember not to adjust for them (see section 'Have they determined whether their groups are comparable, and, if necessary, adjusted for baseline differences?').
3. Do not test your data to see if they are normally distributed. If you do, you might be stuck with non-parametric tests, which aren't as much fun (see section 'What sort of data have they got, and have they used appropriate statistical tests?').
4. Ignore all withdrawals ('drop outs') and non-responders, so the analysis only concerns subjects who fully complied with treatment (see section 'Were preliminary statistical questions addressed?').
5. Always assume that you can plot one set of data against another and calculate an 'r-value' (Pearson correlation coefficient) (see section 'Has correlation been distinguished from regression, and has the correlation coefficient ('r-value') been calculated and interpreted correctly?'), and that a 'significant' r-value proves causation (see section 'Have assumptions been made about the nature and direction of causality?').
6. If outliers (points that lie a long way from the others on your graph) are messing up your calculations, just rub them out. But if outliers are helping your case, even if they appear to be spurious results, leave them in (see section 'Were 'outliers' analysed with both common sense and appropriate statistical adjustments?').
7. If the confidence intervals of your result overlap zero difference between the groups, leave them out of your report. Better still, mention them briefly in the text but don't draw them in on the graph and ignore them when drawing your conclusions (see section 'Have confidence intervals been calculated, and do the authors' conclusions reflect them?').
8. If the difference between two groups becomes significant 4.5 months into a 6-month trial, stop the trial and start writing up. Alternatively if at 6 months, the results are 'nearly significant', extend the trial for another 3 weeks (see section 'Have the data been analysed according to the original study protocol?').
9. If your results prove uninteresting, ask the computer to go back and see if any particular sub-groups behaved differently. You might find that your

intervention worked after all in Chinese women aged 52–61 (see section 'Have the data been analysed according to the original study protocol?').

10. If analysing your data the way you plan to does not give the result you wanted, run the figures through a selection of other tests (see section 'If the statistical tests in the paper are obscure, why have the authors chosen to use them, and have they included a reference?').

Have the authors set the scene correctly?

Have they determined whether their groups are comparable, and, if necessary, adjusted for baseline differences?

Most comparative clinical trials include either a table or a paragraph in the text showing the baseline characteristics of the groups being studied (i.e. their characteristics *before* the trial or observational study was begun). Such a table should demonstrate that both the intervention and control groups are similar in terms of age and sex distribution and key prognostic variables (such as the average size of a cancerous lump). If there are important differences in these baseline characteristics, even though these may be due to chance, it can pose a challenge to your interpretation of results. In this situation, you can carry out certain adjustments to try to allow for these differences and hence strengthen your argument. To find out how to make such adjustments, see the relevant section in any of the mainstream biostatistics textbooks – but don't try to memorise the formulae!

What sort of data have they got, and have they used appropriate statistical tests?

Numbers are often used to label the properties of things. We can assign a number to represent our height, weight and so on. For properties like these, the measurements can be treated as actual numbers. We can, for example, calculate the average weight and height of a group of people by averaging the measurements. But consider a different example, in which we use numbers to label the property 'city of origin', where 1, London, 2, Manchester, 3, Birmingham and so on. We could still calculate the average of these numbers for a particular sample of cases but the result would be meaningless. The same would apply if we labelled the property 'liking for x', with 1, not at all, 2, a bit and 3, a lot. Again, we could calculate the 'average liking' but the numerical result would be uninterpretable unless we knew that the difference between 'not at all' and 'a bit' was exactly the same as the difference between 'a bit' and 'a lot'.

The statistical tests used in medical papers are generally classified as either parametric (i.e. they assume that the data were sampled from a particular form of distribution, such as a normal distribution) or non-parametric (i.e. they do not assume that the data were sampled from a particular type of distribution).

The non-parametric tests focus on the *rank order* of the values (which one is the smallest, which one comes next, etc.), and ignore the absolute differences between them. As you might imagine, statistical significance is more difficult to demonstrate with rank order tests (indeed, some statisticians are cynical about the value of the latter), and this tempts researchers to use statistics such as the r-value (see section 'Has correlation been distinguished from regression, and has the correlation coefficient ("r-value") been calculated and interpreted correctly?') inappropriately. Not only is the r-value (parametric) easier to calculate than an equivalent rank order statistic such as Spearman's ρ (pronounced 'rho') but it is also much more likely to give (apparently) significant results. Unfortunately, it will also give an entirely spurious and misleading estimate of the significance of the result, unless the data are appropriate to the test being used. More examples of parametric tests and their rank order equivalents (if present) are given in Table 5.1.

Another consideration is the shape of the distribution from which the data were sampled. When I was at school, my class plotted the amount of pocket money received against the number of children receiving that amount. The results formed a histogram the same shape as in Figure 5.1 – a 'normal' distribution. (The term *normal* refers to the shape of the graph and is used because many biological phenomena show this pattern of distribution.) Some biological variables such as body weight show *skew* distribution, as shown in Figure 5.2. (Figure 5.2, in fact, shows a negative skew, whereas body weight would be positively skewed. The average adult male body weight is around 80 kg and people exist who are 160 kg but nobody weighs less than nothing, so the graph cannot possibly be symmetrical.)

Non-normal (skewed) data can sometimes be *transformed* to give a normal-shape graph by plotting the logarithm of the skewed variable or performing some other mathematical transformation (such as square root or reciprocal). Some data, however, cannot be transformed into a smooth pattern, and the significance of this is discussed subsequently. Deciding whether data are normally distributed is not an academic exercise, because it will determine what type of statistical tests to use. For example, linear regression (see section 'Correlation, regression and causation') will give misleading results unless the points on the scatter graph form a particular distribution about the regression line – that is, the residuals (the perpendicular distance from each point to the line) should themselves be normally distributed. Transforming data to achieve a normal distribution (if this is indeed achievable) is not cheating.

Table 5.1 Some commonly used statistical tests

Parametric test	Example of equivalent non-parametric (rank order) test	Purpose of test	Example
Two sample (unpaired) t-test	Mann–Whitney U-test.	Compares two independent samples drawn from the same population.	To compare girls' heights with boys' heights.
One-sample (paired) t-test	Wilcoxon matched-pairs test.	Compares two sets of observations on a single sample (tests the hypothesis that the mean difference between two measurements is zero).	To compare weight of infants before and after a feed.
One-way analysis of variance using total sum of squares (e.g. F-test)	Analysis of variance by ranks (e.g. Kruskall–Wallis test).	Effectively, a generalisation of the paired t-test or Wilcoxon matched-pairs test where three or more sets of observations are made on a single sample.	To determine whether plasma glucose level is higher 1, 2 or 3 h after a meal.
Two-way analysis of variance	Two-way analysis of variance by ranks.	As mentioned, but tests the influence (and interaction) of two different covariates.	In the earlier example, to determine if the results differ in men and women.
No direct equivalent	χ^2 test	Tests the null hypothesis that the proportions of variables estimated from two (or more) independent samples are the same.	To assess whether acceptance into medical school is more likely if the applicant was born in the UK.
No direct equivalent	McNemar's test	Tests the null hypothesis that the proportions estimated from a paired sample are the same.	To compare the sensitivity and specificity of two different diagnostic tests when applied to the same sample.

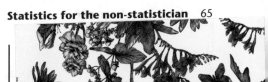

Product moment correlation coefficient (Pearson's r)	Spearman's rank correlation coefficient (ρ).	Assesses the *strength* of the straight-line association between two continuous variables.	To assess whether and to what extent plasma HbA1 level is related to plasma triglyceride level in diabetic patients.
Regression by least-squares method	No direct equivalent	Describes the numerical relation between two quantitative variables, allowing one value to be predicted from the other.	To see how peak expiratory flow rate varies with height.
Multiple regression by least-squares method	No direct equivalent	Describes the numerical relation between a dependent variable and several predictor variables (covariates).	To determine whether and to what extent a person's age, body fat and sodium intake determine their blood pressure.

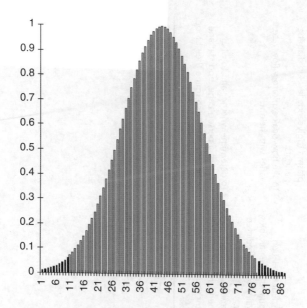

Figure 5.1 Example of a normal curve.

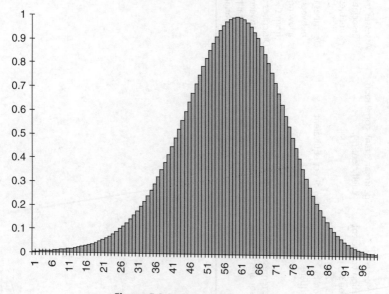

Figure 5.2 Example of a skew curve.

It simply ensures that data values are given appropriate emphasis in assessing the overall effect. Using tests based on the normal distribution to analyse non-normally distributed data is very definitely cheating.

If the statistical tests in the paper are obscure, why have the authors chosen to use them, and have they included a reference?

There sometimes seems to be an infinite number of possible statistical tests. In fact, most basic clinical studies can be analysed using a formulary of about a dozen. The rest are small-print, and should be reserved for special indications. If the paper you are reading appears to describe a standard set of data that have been collected in a standard way, but the test used is unpronounceable and not listed in a basic statistics textbook, you should smell a rat. The authors should, in such circumstances, state why they have used this test, and give a reference (with page numbers) for a definitive description of it.

Have the data been analysed according to the original study protocol?

Even if you are not interested in the statistical justification, common sense should tell you why points 8 and 9 in Box 5.2 at the end of this chapter amount to serious cheating. If you trawl for long enough, you will inevitably find some category of participants who appear to have done particularly well or badly. However, each time you look to see if a particular subgroup is different from the rest you greatly increase the likelihood that you will eventually find one that appears to be so, even though the difference is entirely due to chance.

Box 5.2 Tests for causation (see Reference [14])

1. Is there evidence from true experiments in humans?
2. Is the association strong?
3. Is the association consistent from study to study?
4. Is the temporal relationship appropriate (i.e. did the postulated cause precede the postulated effect)?
5. Is there a dose–response gradient (i.e. does more of the postulated effect follow more of the postulated cause)?
6. Does the association make epidemiological sense?
7. Does the association make biological sense?
8. Is the association specific?
9. Is the association analogous to a previously proven causal association?

Similarly, if you play coin toss with someone, no matter how far you fall behind, there will come a time when you are one ahead. Most people would agree that to stop the game then would not be a fair way to play. So it is with research. If you make it inevitable that you will (eventually) obtain an apparently positive result you will also make it inevitable that you will be misleading yourself about the justice of your case. Terminating an intervention trial prematurely for ethical reasons when participants in one arm are faring particularly badly is different, and is discussed elsewhere [8].

Going back and raking over your data to look for 'interesting' results (retrospective subgroup analysis or, more colloquially, data dredging) can lead to false conclusions [9, 10]. In an early study on the use of aspirin in the prevention of stroke in predisposed patients, the results showed a significant effect in both sexes combined, and a retrospective subgroup analysis appeared to show that the effect was confined to men [11]. This conclusion led to aspirin being withheld from women for many years until the results of other studies (including a large meta-analysis [12]) showed this subgroup effect to be spurious.

This and other examples are given in a paper by Oxman and Guyatt [13], 'A consumer's guide to subgroup analysis', which reproduces a useful checklist for deciding whether apparent differences in subgroup response are real.

Paired data, tails and outliers

Were paired tests performed on paired data?

Students often find it difficult to decide whether to use a paired or unpaired statistical test to analyse their data. There is, in fact, no great mystery about this. If you measure something twice on each participant (e.g. lying and standing blood pressure), you will probably be interested not just in the average difference in lying versus standing blood pressure in the entire sample, but in how much each individual's blood pressure changes with position. In this situation, you have what are called *paired* data, because each measurement beforehand is paired with a measurement afterwards.

In this example, it is having the same person on both occasions that makes the pairings, but there are other possibilities (e.g. any two measurements made of bed occupancy of the same hospital ward). In these situations, it is likely that the two sets of values will be significantly correlated (e.g. my blood pressure next week is likely to be closer to my blood pressure last week than to the blood pressure of a randomly selected adult last week). In other words, we would expect two randomly selected 'paired' values to be closer to each other than two randomly selected 'unpaired' values. Unless we allow for this, by carrying out the appropriate 'paired' sample tests, we can end up with a biased estimate of the significance of our results.

Was a two-tailed test performed whenever the effect of an intervention could conceivably be a negative one?

The concept of a test with tails always has me thinking of devils or snakes, which I guess just reflects my aversion to statistics. In fact, the term *tail* refers to the extremes of the distribution – the dark areas in Figure 5.1. Let's say that graph represents the diastolic blood pressures of a group of individuals of which a random sample are about to be put on a low-sodium diet. If a low-sodium diet has a significant lowering effect on blood pressure, subsequent blood pressure measurements on these participants would be more likely to lie within the left-hand 'tail' of the graph. Hence, we would analyse the data with statistical tests designed to show whether unusually low readings in this patient sample were likely to have arisen by chance.

But on what grounds may we assume that a low-sodium diet could only conceivably put blood pressure down, but could never put it *up*? Even if there are valid physiological reasons why that might be the case in this particular example, it is certainly not good science always to assume that you know the *direction* of the effect that your intervention will have. A new drug intended to relieve nausea might actually exacerbate it; and an educational leaflet intended to reduce anxiety might increase it. Hence, your statistical analysis should, in general, test the hypothesis that either high *or* low values in your dataset have arisen by chance. In the language of the statisticians, this means you need a two-tailed test unless you have very convincing evidence that the difference can only be in one direction.

Were 'outliers' analysed with both common sense and appropriate statistical adjustments?

Unexpected results may reflect idiosyncrasies in the participant (e.g. unusual metabolism), errors in measurement (e.g. faulty equipment), errors in interpretation (e.g. misreading a meter reading), or errors in calculation (e.g. misplaced decimal points). Only the first of these is a 'real' result that deserves to be included in the analysis. A result that is many orders of magnitude away from the others is less likely to be genuine, but it may be. A few years ago, while doing a research project, I measured a number of different hormone levels in about 30 participants. One participant's growth hormone levels came back about a hundred times higher than everyone else's. I assumed this was a transcription error, so I moved the decimal point two places to the left. Some weeks later, I met the technician who had analysed the specimens and he asked 'Whatever happened to that chap with acromegaly?'

Statistically correcting for outliers (e.g. to modify their effect on the overall result) is quite a sophisticated statistical manoeuvre. If you are interested, try the relevant section in your favourite statistics textbook.

Correlation, regression and causation

Has correlation been distinguished from regression, and has the correlation coefficient ('r-value') been calculated and interpreted correctly?

For many non-statisticians, the terms *correlation* and *regression* are synonymous, and refer vaguely to a mental image of a scatter graph with dots sprinkled messily along a diagonal line sprouting from the intercept of the axes. You would be right in assuming that if two things are not correlated, it will be meaningless to attempt a regression. But regression and correlation are both precise statistical terms that serve different functions [2].

The r-value (or to give it its official name, 'Pearson's product–moment correlation coefficient') is among the most overused statistical instruments in the book. Strictly speaking, the r-value is not valid unless certain criteria, as given here, are fulfilled.

1. The data (or, more accurately, the population from which the data are drawn) should be normally distributed. If they are not, non-parametric tests of correlation should be used instead (see Table 5.1).
2. The two variables should be structurally independent (i.e. one should not be forced to vary with the other). If they are not, a paired *t* or other paired test should be used instead.
3. Only a single pair of measurements should be made on each participant, as the measurements made on successive participants need to be statistically independent of each other if we are to end up with unbiased estimates of the population parameters of interest.
4. Every r-value should be accompanied by a p-value, which expresses how likely an association of this strength would be to have arisen by chance (see section 'Have 'p-values' been calculated and interpreted appropriately?'), or a confidence interval, which expresses the range within which the 'true' R-value is likely to lie (see section 'Have confidence intervals been calculated, and do the authors' conclusions reflect them?'). (Note that lower case 'r' represents the correlation coefficient of the sample, whereas upper case 'R' represents the correlation coefficient of the entire population.)

Remember, too, that even if the r-value is an appropriate value to calculate from a set of data, it does not tell you whether the relationship, however strong, is causal (see subsequent text).

The term *regression* refers to a mathematical *equation* that allows one variable (the *target* variable) to be predicted from another (the *independent* variable). Regression, then, implies a direction of influence, although as the next section will argue, it does not prove causality. In the case of multiple regression, a far more complex mathematical equation (which, thankfully, usually remains the secret of the computer that calculated it) allows the target variable to be predicted from two or more independent variables (often known as *covariables*).

The simplest regression equation, which you may remember from your school days, is $y = a + bx$, where y is the dependent variable (plotted on the vertical axis), x is the independent variable (plotted on the horizontal axis), a is the y-intercept and b is a constant. Not many biological variables can be predicted with such a simple equation. The weight of a group of people, for example, varies with their height, but not in a linear way. In the first edition of this book, I gave the example 'I am twice as tall as my son and three times his weight, but although I am four times as tall as my newborn nephew I am much more than six times his weight'. Both son and nephew now tower over me, but the example will hold. Weight probably varies more closely with the square of someone's height than with height itself, so a quadratic rather than a linear regression would be more appropriate.

Even when you have fed sufficient height–weight data into a computer for it to calculate the regression equation that best predicts a person's weight from their height, your predictions would still be pretty poor, as weight and height are not all that closely *correlated*. There are other things that influence weight in addition to height, and we could, to illustrate the principle of multiple regression, enter data on age, sex, daily calorie intake and physical activity level into the computer and ask it how much each of these covariables contributes to the overall equation (or model).

The elementary principles described here, particularly the numbered points earlier, should help you spot whether correlation and regression are being used correctly in the paper you are reading. A more detailed discussion on the subject can be found in statistical textbooks listed at the end of this chapter [5–7], and in the fourth article in the Basic Statistics for Clinicians series [2].

Have assumptions been made about the nature and direction of causality?

Remember the ecological fallacy: just because a town has a large number of unemployed people and a very high crime rate, it does not necessarily follow that the unemployed are committing the crimes! In other words, the presence of an *association* between A and B tells you nothing at all about either the presence or the direction of causality. In order to demonstrate that A has *caused* B (rather than B causing A, or A and B both being caused by C), you need more than a correlation coefficient. Box 5.1 gives some criteria, originally developed by Sir Austin Bradford Hill [14], which should be met before assuming causality.

Probability and confidence

Have 'p-values' been calculated and interpreted appropriately?

One of the first values a student of statistics learns to calculate is the p-value – that is the probability that any particular outcome would have arisen by chance. Standard scientific practice, which is essentially arbitrary, usually deems a p-value of less than one in twenty (expressed as $p < 0.05$, and equivalent to a betting odds of twenty to one) as 'statistically significant', and a p-value of less than one in a hundred ($p < 0.01$) as 'statistically highly significant'.

By definition, then, one chance association in twenty (this must be around one major published result per journal issue) will appear to be significant when it isn't, and one in a hundred will appear highly significant when it is really what my children call a 'fluke'. Hence, if the researchers have made multiple comparisons, they ought to make a correction to try to allow for this. The most widely known procedure for doing this is probably the Bonferroni test (described in most standard statistical textbooks), although a reviewer of earlier editions of this book described this as 'far too severe' and offered several others. Rather than speculate on tests that I don't personally understand, I recommend asking a statistician's advice if the paper you are reading makes multiple comparisons.

A result in the statistically significant range ($p < 0.05$ or $p < 0.01$ depending on what you have chosen as the cutoff) suggests that the authors should reject the null hypothesis (i.e. the hypothesis that there is no real difference between two groups). But as I have argued earlier (see section 'Were preliminary statistical questions addressed?'), a p-value in the non-significant range tells you that *either* there is no difference between the groups *or* there were too few participants to demonstrate such a difference if it existed. It does not tell you which.

The p-value has a further limitation. Guyatt and colleagues conclude thus, in the first article of their 'Basic Statistics for Clinicians' series on hypothesis testing using p-values.

Why use a single cut-off point [for statistical significance] when the choice of such a point is arbitrary? Why make the question of whether a treatment is effective a dichotomy (a yes-no decision) when it would be more appropriate to view it as a continuum? [1].

For this, we need confidence intervals, which are considered next.

Have confidence intervals been calculated, and do the authors' conclusions reflect them?

A confidence interval, which a good statistician can calculate on the result of just about any statistical test (the *t*-test, the *r*-value, the absolute risk reduction (ARR), the number needed to treat and the sensitivity, specificity and other key features of a diagnostic test), allows you to estimate for both 'positive' trials (those that show a statistically significant difference between two arms of the trial) and 'negative' ones (those that appear to show no difference), whether the strength of the evidence is *strong* or *weak*, and whether the study is *definitive* (i.e. obviates the need for further similar studies). The calculation of confidence intervals has been covered with great clarity in the classic book 'Statistics with Confidence' [15], and their interpretation has been covered by Guyatt and colleagues [4].

If you repeated the same clinical trial hundreds of times, you would not obtain exactly the same result each time. But, *on average*, you would establish a particular level of difference (or lack of difference!) between the two arms of the trial. In 90% of the trials, the difference between two arms would lie within certain broad limits, and in 95% of the trials, it would lie between certain, even broader, limits.

Now, if, as is usually the case, you only conducted one trial, how do you know how close the result is to the 'real' difference between the groups? The answer is you don't. But by calculating, say, the 95% confidence interval around your result, you will be able to say that there is a 95% chance that the 'real' difference lies between these two limits. The sentence to look for in a paper should read something like this one.

In a trial of the treatment of heart failure, 33% of the patients randomised to ACE inhibitors died, whereas 38% of those randomised to hydralazine and nitrates died. The point estimate of the difference between the groups [the best single estimate of the benefit in lives saved from the use of an ACE inhibitor] is 5%. The 95% confidence interval around this difference is −1.2% to +12%.

More likely, the results would be expressed in the following shorthand.

The ACE inhibitor group had a 5% (95% CI −1.2 + 12) higher survival.

In this particular example, the 95% confidence interval overlaps zero difference and, if we were expressing the result as a dichotomy (i.e. is the hypothesis
'proven' or 'disproven'?), we would classify it as a negative trial. Yet, as Guyatt
and colleagues argue, there *probably* is a real difference, and it *probably* lies
closer to 5% than either −1.2% or +12%. A more useful conclusion from these
results is that 'all else being equal, an angiotensin-converting enzyme (ACE)
inhibitor is probably the appropriate choice for patients with heart failure, but
the strength of that inference is weak' [4].

As section 'Ten questions to ask about a paper that claims to validate a diagnostic or screening test' argues, the larger the trial (or the larger the pooled
results of several trials), the narrower the confidence interval – and, therefore,
the more likely the result is to be definitive.

In interpreting 'negative' trials, one important thing you need to know is
'would a much larger trial be likely to show a significant benefit?'. To answer
this question, look at the *upper* 95% confidence interval of the result. There
is only one chance in forty (i.e. a $2^1/_2$% chance, as the other $2^1/_2$% of extreme
results will lie below the *lower* 95% confidence interval) that the real result
will be this much or more. Now ask yourself: 'Would this level of difference
be *clinically* significant?', and if it wouldn't, you can classify the trial as not
only negative but also definitive. If, on the other hand, the upper 95% confidence interval represented a clinically significant level of difference between
the groups, the trial may be negative but it is also non-definitive.

Until fairly recently, the use of confidence intervals was relatively
uncommon in medical papers. Fortunately, most trials in journals that follow
Consolidated Standards of Reporting Trials (CONSORT) guidelines (see
section 'Randomised controlled trials') now include these routinely, but even
so, many authors do not interpret their confidence intervals correctly. You
should check carefully in the discussion section to see whether the authors
have correctly concluded (i) whether and to what extent their trial supported
their hypothesis, and (ii) whether any further studies need to be done.

The bottom line

Have the authors expressed the effects of an intervention in terms of the likely benefit or harm that an individual patient can expect?

It is all very well to say that a particular intervention produces a 'statistically
significant difference' in outcome but if I were being asked to take a new

medicine I would want to know how much better my chances would be (in terms of any particular outcome) than they would be if I didn't take it. Three simple calculations (and I promise you they *are* simple: if you can add, subtract, multiply and divide you will be able to follow this section) will enable you to answer this question objectively and in a way which means something to the non-statistician. The calculations are the relative risk reduction, the ARR and the number needed to treat.

To illustrate these concepts, and to persuade you that you need to know about them, let me tell you about a survey that Fahey and his colleagues [16] conducted a few years ago. They wrote to 182 board members of district health authorities in England (all of whom would be in some way responsible for making important health service decisions), and put the following data to them about four different rehabilitation programmes for heart attack victims. They asked which one they would prefer to fund.

Programme A – which reduced the rate of deaths by 20%.

Programme B – which produced an absolute reduction in deaths of 3%.

Programme C – which increased patients' survival rate from 84% to 87%.

Programme D – which meant that 31 people needed to enter the programme to avoid one death.

Of the 140 board members who responded, only three spotted that all four 'programmes' in fact related to the same set of results. The other 137 participants all selected one of the programmes in preference to one of the others, thus revealing (as well as their own ignorance) the need for better basic training in epidemiology for healthcare policymakers. In fact, 'Programme A' is the relative risk reduction; 'Programme B' is the ARR; 'Programme C' is another way of expressing the ARR and 'Programme D' is the number needed to treat.

Let's continue with this example, which Fahey and colleagues reproduced from a study by Yusuf and colleagues [17]. I have expressed the figures as a two by two table giving details of which treatment the patients received in their randomised trial, and whether they were dead or alive 10 years later (Table 5.2).

Table 5.2 Data from a trial of medical therapy versus coronary artery bypass grafting after heart attack [16, 17]

Treatment	Outcome at 10 years Dead alive	Total number of patients randomised in each group
Medical therapy	404 921	1325
CABG	350 974	1324

Simple maths tells you that patients on medical therapy have a $404/1325 = 0.305$ or 30.5% chance of being dead at 10 years. This is the *absolute risk* of death for the control (medical therapy) group: let's call it x. Patients randomised to coronary artery bypass grafting (CABG) have a $350/1324 = 0.264$ or 26.4% chance of being dead at 10 years. This is the absolute risk of death for the intervention (CABG) group: let's call it y.

The *relative risk* of death in CABG patients compared with medical intervention controls – is y/x or $0.264/0.305 = 0.87$ (87%).

The *relative risk reduction* – that is, the amount by which the risk of death is reduced in the CABG group compared to the control group – is $100 - 87\%$ $(1 - y/x) = 13\%$.

The *ARR* (or risk difference) – that is, the absolute amount by which CABG reduces the risk of death at 10 years – is $30.5 - 26.4\% = 4.1\%$ (0.041).

The *number needed to treat* – that is, how many patients need a CABG in order to prevent, on average, one death by 10 years – is the reciprocal of the ARR, $1/ARR = 1/0.041 = 24$.

The general formulae for calculating these 'bottom line' effects of an intervention are reproduced in Appendix 2, and for a discussion on which of these values is most useful in which circumstances, see Jaeschke and colleagues' article in the 'Basic Statistics for Clinicians' series [3].

Summary

It is possible to be seriously misled by taking the statistical competence (and/or the intellectual honesty) of authors for granted. Statistics can be an intimidating science, and understanding its finer points often calls for expert help. But I hope that this chapter has shown you that the statistics used in most medical research papers can be evaluated – at least up to a point – by the non-expert using a simple checklist such as that in Appendix 1. In addition, you might like to check the paper you are reading (or writing) against the common errors given in Box 5.2.

References

1 Guyatt G, Jaeschke R, Heddle N, et al. Basic statistics for clinicians: 1. Hypothesis testing. CMAJ: Canadian Medical Association Journal 1995;**152**(1):27.
2 Guyatt G, Walter S, Shannon H, et al. Basic statistics for clinicians: 4. Correlation and regression. CMAJ: Canadian Medical Association Journal 1995;**152**(4):497.
3 Jaeschke R, Guyatt G, Shannon H, et al. Basic statistics for clinicians: 3. Assessing the effects of treatment: measures of association. CMAJ: Canadian Medical Association Journal 1995;**152**(3):351.

4 Guyatt G, Jaeschke R, Heddle N, et al. Basic statistics for clinicians: 2. Interpreting study results: confidence intervals. CMAJ: Canadian Medical Association Journal 1995;**152**(2):169.

5 Norman GR, Streiner DL. *Biostatistics: the bare essentials.* USA: PMPH-USA, 2007.

6 Bowers D. *Medical statistics from scratch: an introduction for health professionals.* Oxford: John Wiley & Sons, 2008.

7 Bland M. *An introduction to medical statistics.* Oxford: Oxford University Press, 2000.

8 Pocock SJ. When (not) to stop a clinical trial for benefit. JAMA: The Journal of the American Medical Association 2005;**294**(17):2228–30.

9 Cuff A. Sources of Bias in Clinical Trials. 2013. http://applyingcriticality.wordpress.com/2013/06/19/sources-of-bias-in-clinical-trials/ (accessed 26th June 2013).

10 Delgado-Rodríguez M, Llorca J. Bias. Journal of Epidemiology and Community Health 2004;**58**(8):635–41 doi: 10.1136/jech.2003.008466.

11 Group CCS. A randomized trial of aspirin and sulfinpyrazone in threatened stroke. The New England Journal of Medicine 1978;**299**(2):53–9.

12 Antiplatelet Trialists' Collaboration. Secondary prevention of vascular disease by prolonged antiplatelet treatment. British Medical Journal (Clinical Research Edition) 1988;**296**(6618):320.

13 Oxman AD, Guyatt GH. A consumer's guide to subgroup analyses. Annals of Internal Medicine 1992;**116**(1):78–84.

14 Hill AB. The environment and disease: association or causation? Proceedings of the Royal Society of Medicine 1965;**58**(5):295.

15 Altman DG, Machin D, Bryant TN, et al. *Statistics with confidence: confidence intervals and statistical guidelines.* London: BMJ Books, 2000.

16 Fahey T, Griffiths S, Peters T. Evidence based purchasing: understanding results of clinical trials and systematic reviews. BMJ: British Medical Journal 1995;**311**(7012):1056–9.

17 Yusuf S, Zucker D, Passamani E, et al. Effect of coronary artery bypass graft surgery on survival: overview of 10-year results from randomised trials by the Coronary Artery Bypass Graft Surgery Trialists Collaboration. The Lancet 1994;**344**(8922):563–70.

Chapter 6 Papers that report trials of drug treatments and other simple interventions

'Evidence' and marketing

This chapter is about evaluating evidence from clinical trials, and most of that evidence is about drugs. If you are a clinical doctor, nurse practitioner or pharmacist (i.e. if you prescribe or dispense drugs), the pharmaceutical industry is interested in you, and spends a proportion of its multi-million pound annual advertising budget trying to influence you (see Box 6.1) [1]. Even if you are a mere patient, the industry can now target you directly through direct-to-consumer-advertising (DTCA) [2]. When I wrote the first edition of this book in 1995, the standard management of vaginal thrush (*Candida* infection) was for a doctor to prescribe clotrimazole pessaries. By the time the second edition was published in 2001, these pessaries were available over the counter in pharmacies. For the past 10 years, clotrimazole has been advertised on prime-time TV – thankfully after the nine o'clock watershed – and more recently the manufacturers of this and other powerful drugs are advertising via the Internet and social media [3]. In case you were wondering, such advertising subtly tends to place more emphasis on benefits than risks [4].

The most effective way of changing the prescribing habits of a clinician is via a personal representative (known to most of us in the UK as the 'drug rep' and to our North American colleagues as the 'detailer'), who travels round with a briefcase full of 'evidence' in support of his or her wares [5]. Indeed, as I discuss in more detail in Chapters 14 and 15, the evidence-based medicine movement has learnt a lot from the drug industry in recent years about changing the behaviour of physicians, and now uses the same sophisticated techniques of persuasion in what is known as *academic detailing* of individual health professionals [6]. Interestingly, DTCA often works by harnessing the persuasive power of the patient – who effectively becomes an unpaid 'rep'

How to Read a Paper: The Basics of Evidence-Based Medicine, Fifth Edition. Trisha Greenhalgh.
© 2014 John Wiley & Sons, Ltd. Published 2014 by John Wiley & Sons, Ltd.

Box 6.1 Ten tips for the pharmaceutical industry: how to present your product in the best light

1. Think up a plausible physiological mechanism why the drug works, and become slick at presenting it. Preferably, find a surrogate endpoint that is heavily influenced by the drug, although it may not be strictly valid (see section 'Making decisions about therapy');

2. When designing clinical trials, select a patient population, clinical features and trial length that reflect the maximum possible response to the drug.

3. If possible, compare your product only with placebos. If you must compare it with a competitor, make sure the latter is given at sub-therapeutic dose.

4. Include the results of pilot studies in the figures for definitive studies, so it looks like more patients have been randomised than is actually the case.

5. Omit mention of any trial that had a fatality or serious adverse drug reaction in the treatment group. If possible, don't publish such studies.

6. Have your graphics department maximise the visual impact of your message. It helps not to label the axes of graphs or say whether scales are linear or logarithmic. Make sure you do not show individual patient data or confidence intervals.

7. Become master of the hanging comparative ('better' – but better than what?).

8. Invert the standard hierarchy of evidence so that anecdote takes precedence over randomised trials and meta-analyses.

9. Name at least three local opinion leaders who use the drug, and offer 'starter packs' for the doctor to try.

10. Present a 'cost-effectiveness' analysis which shows that your product, even though more expensive than its competitor, 'actually works out cheaper' (see section 'The great guidelines debate').

for the pharmaceutical industry. If you think you'd be able to resist a patient more easily than a real rep, you're probably wrong – one randomised controlled trial showed a highly significant effect of patient power on doctors' prescribing following DTCA for antidepressants [7].

Before you agree to meet a rep (or a patient armed with material from a newspaper article or DTCA website), remind yourself of some basic rules of research design. As sections 'Cohort studies' and 'Cross-sectional surveys' argued, questions about the benefits of therapy should ideally be addressed with randomised controlled trials. But preliminary questions about pharmacokinetics (i.e. how the drug behaves while it is getting to its site of action), particularly those relating to bioavailability, require a straight dosing experiment in healthy (and, if ethical and practicable, sick) volunteers.

Common (and probably trivial) adverse drug reactions may be picked up, and their incidence quantified, in the randomised controlled trials undertaken to demonstrate the drug's efficacy. But rare (and usually more serious) adverse drug reactions require both pharmacovigilance surveys (collection of data prospectively on patients receiving a newly licensed drug) and case–control studies (see section 'Cohort studies') to establish association. Ideally, individual rechallenge experiments (where the patient who has had a reaction considered to be caused by the drug is given the drug again in carefully supervised circumstances) should be performed to establish causation [8].

Pharmaceutical reps do not tell nearly as many lies as they used to (drug marketing has become an altogether more sophisticated science), but as Goldacre [9] has shown in his book 'Bad Pharma', they still provide information that is at best selective and at worst overtly biased. It often helps their case, for example, to present the results of uncontrolled trials and express them in terms of before-and-after differences in a particular outcome measure. Reference to section 'Cross-sectional surveys' and the literature on placebo effects [10, 11] should remind you why uncontrolled before-and-after studies are the stuff of teenage magazines, not hard science.

Dr Herxheimer, who edited the *Drug and Therapeutics Bulletin* for many years, undertook a survey of 'references' cited in advertisements for pharmaceutical products in the leading UK medical journals. He tells me that a high proportion of such references cite 'data on file', and many more refer to publications written, edited and published entirely by the industry. Evidence from these sources has sometimes (although by no means invariably) been shown to be of lower scientific quality than that which appears in independent, peer-reviewed journals. And let's face it, if you worked for a drug company that had made a major scientific breakthrough you would probably submit your findings to a publication such as the *Lancet* or the *New England Journal of Medicine* before publishing them in-house. In other words, you don't need to 'trash' papers about drug trials *because* of where they have been published, but you do need to look closely at the methods and statistical analysis of such trials.

Making decisions about therapy

Sackett and colleagues [8], in their book '*Clinical epidemiology – a basic science for clinical medicine*', argue that before starting a patient on a drug, the doctor should:

(a) identify *for this patient* the ultimate objective of treatment (cure, prevention of recurrence, limitation of functional disability, prevention of later complications, reassurance, palliation, symptomatic relief, etc.);

(b) select the *most appropriate* treatment using all available evidence (this includes addressing the question of whether the patient needs to take any drug at all);

(c) specify the *treatment target* (how will you know when to stop treatment, change its intensity or switch to some other treatment?).

For example, in the treatment of high blood pressure, the doctor might decide that:

(a) the *ultimate objective of treatment* is to prevent (further) target organ damage to brain, eye, heart, kidney, and so on (and thereby prevent death);

(b) the *choice of specific treatment* is between the various classes of antihypertensive drugs selected on the basis of randomised, placebo-controlled and comparative trials – as well as between non-drug treatments such as salt restriction; and

(c) the *treatment target* might be a Phase V diastolic blood pressure (right arm, sitting) of less than 90 mmHg, or as close to that as tolerable in the face of drug side effects.

If these three steps are not followed (as is often the case – e.g. in terminal care), therapeutic chaos can result. In a veiled slight on surrogate endpoints, Sackett and his team remind us that the choice of specific therapy should be determined by evidence of what *does* work, and not on what *seems* to work or *ought* to work. 'Today's therapy', they warn, 'when derived from biologic facts or uncontrolled clinical experience, may become tomorrow's bad joke' [8].

Surrogate endpoints

I have not included this section solely because it is a particular hobby horse of mine. If you are a practising (and non-academic) clinician, your main contact with published papers may well be through what gets fed to you by a 'drug rep'. The pharmaceutical industry is a slick player at the surrogate endpoint game, and I make no apology for labouring the point that such outcome measures must be evaluated very carefully.

I will define a surrogate endpoint as '*a variable which is relatively easily measured and which predicts a rare or distant outcome of either a toxic stimulus (e.g. pollutant) or a therapeutic intervention (e.g. drug, surgical procedure, piece of advice), but which is not itself a direct measure of either harm or clinical benefit*'. The growing interest in surrogate endpoints in medical research reflects two important features of their use.

- They can considerably reduce the *sample size*, *duration* and, therefore, *cost*, of clinical trials.
- They can allow treatments to be assessed in situations where the use of primary outcomes would be excessively *invasive* or *unethical*.

In the evaluation of pharmaceutical products, commonly used surrogate endpoints include

- pharmacokinetic measurements (e.g. concentration–time curves of a drug or its active metabolite in the bloodstream);
- *in vitro* (i.e. laboratory) measures such as the mean inhibitory concentration (MIC) of an antimicrobial against a bacterial culture on agar;
- macroscopic appearance of tissues (e.g. gastric erosion seen at endoscopy);
- change in levels of (alleged) 'biological markers of disease' (e.g. microalbuminuria in the measurement of diabetic kidney disease);
- radiological appearance (e.g. shadowing on a chest X-ray – or in a more contemporary setting, functional magnetic resonance imaging).

Surrogate endpoints have a number of drawbacks. First, a change in the surrogate endpoint does not itself answer the essential preliminary questions: 'what is the objective of treatment in this patient?' and 'what, according to valid and reliable research studies, is the best available treatment for this condition?'. Second, the surrogate endpoint may not closely reflect the treatment target – in other words, it may not be valid or reliable. Third, the use of a surrogate endpoint has the same limitations as the use of any other *single* measure of the success or failure of therapy – it ignores all the other measures! Over-reliance on a single surrogate endpoint as a measure of therapeutic success usually reflects a narrow or naïve clinical perspective.

Finally, surrogate endpoints are often developed in animal models of disease because changes in a specific variable can be measured under controlled conditions in a well-defined population. However, extrapolation of these findings to human disease is liable to be invalid [12].

- In animal studies, the population being studied has fairly uniform biological characteristics and may be genetically inbred.
- Both the tissue and the disease being studied may vary in important characteristics (e.g. susceptibility to the pathogen, rate of cell replication) from the parallel condition in human subjects.
- The animals are kept in a controlled environment, which minimises the influence of lifestyle variables (e.g. diet, exercise, stress) and concomitant medication.
- Giving high doses of chemicals to experimental animals may distort the usual metabolic pathways and thereby give misleading results. Animal species best suited to serve as a surrogate for humans vary for different chemicals.

The ideal features of a surrogate endpoint are shown in Box 6.2. If the 'rep' who is trying to persuade you about the value of the drug cannot justify the endpoints used, you should challenge him or her to produce additional evidence.

If you are interested in pursuing some real examples of surrogate endpoints that led to misleading practices and recommendations, try these.

- The use of ECG findings instead of clinical outcomes (syncope, death) in deciding the efficacy and safety of anti-arrhythmia drugs [13];
- The use of X-ray findings instead of clinical outcomes (pain, loss of function) to monitor the progression of osteoarthritis and the efficacy of disease-modifying drugs [14];

Box 6.2 Ideal features of a surrogate endpoint

1. The surrogate endpoint should be reliable, reproducible, clinically available, easily quantifiable, affordable and exhibit a 'dose–response' effect (i.e. the higher the level of the surrogate endpoint, the greater the probability of disease).
2. It should be a true predictor of disease (or risk of disease) and not merely express exposure to a covariable. The relationship between the surrogate endpoint and the disease should have a biologically plausible explanation.
3. It should be sensitive – that is, a 'positive' result in the surrogate endpoint should pick up all or most patients at increased risk of adverse outcome.
4. It should be specific – that is, a 'negative' result should exclude all or most of those without increased risk of adverse outcome.
5. There should be a precise cut-off between normal and abnormal values.
6. It should have an acceptable positive predictive value – that is, a 'positive' result should always or usually mean that the patient thus identified is at increased risk of adverse outcome (see section 'Ten questions to ask about a paper describing a complex intervention').
7. It should have an acceptable negative predictive value – that is, a 'negative' result should always or usually mean that the patient thus identified is not at increased risk of adverse outcome (see section 'Ten questions to ask about a paper describing a complex intervention').
8. It should be amenable to quality control monitoring.
9. Changes in the surrogate endpoint should rapidly and accurately reflect the response to therapy – in particular, levels should normalise in states of remission or cure.

- The use of albuminuria instead of the overall clinical benefit–harm balance to evaluate the usefulness of dual renin–angiotensin blockade in hypertension [15, 16]. In this example, the intervention was based on a hypothetical argument that blocking the renin–angiotensin pathway at two separate stages would be doubly effective, and the surrogate marker confirmed that this seemed to be the case – but the combination was also doubly effective at producing the potentially fatal side effect of hypokalaemia!

It would be unsporting to suggest that the pharmaceutical industry always develops surrogate endpoints with the deliberate intention of misleading the licensing authorities and health professionals. Surrogate endpoints, as I argued in section "'Evidence" and marketing', have both ethical and economic imperatives. However, the industry does have a vested interest in overstating its case on the strength of these endpoints [9], so use caution when you read a paper whose findings are not based on 'hard patient-relevant outcomes'.

Surrogate endpoints are only one of many ways in which industry-sponsored trials may give a misleading impression of the efficacy of a drug. Other subtle (and not so subtle) influences on research design – such as framing the question in a particular way or selective reporting of findings – have been described in a recent Cochrane review of how industry-sponsored trials tend to favour industry products [17].

What information to expect in a paper describing a randomised controlled trial: the CONSORT statement

Drug trials are an example of a 'simple intervention' – that is, an intervention that is well demarcated (i.e. it's easy to say what the intervention comprises) and lends itself to an 'intervention on' versus 'intervention off' research design. In Chapters 3 and 4, I gave some preliminary advice on assessing the methodological quality of research studies. Here's some more detail. In 1996, an international working group produced a standard checklist, known as *Consolidated Standards of Reporting Trials* (*CONSORT*), for reporting randomised controlled trials in medical journals, and this has now been updated several times, the latest in 2010 [18]. Without doubt, the use of such checklists has increased the quality and consistency of reporting of trials in the medical literature [19]. A checklist based on the CONSORT statement is reproduced in Table 6.1. Please do not try to learn this table off by heart (I certainly couldn't reproduce it myself from memory), but do refer to it if you are asked to critically appraise a paper to which it applies – or if you are planning on doing a randomised trial yourself.

Incidentally, one important way to reduce bias in drug marketing is to ensure that every trial that is *begun* is also written up and *published* [20].

Table 6.1 Checklist for a randomised controlled trial based on the CONSORT statement (see Reference [17])

Title/abstract	Do the title and abstract say how participants were allocated to interventions (e.g., 'random allocation', 'randomised' or 'randomly assigned')?
Introduction	Is the scientific background and rationale for the study adequately explained?
Methods	
Objectives	Were the specific objectives and/or hypothesis to be tested stated explicitly?
Participants and setting	Does the paper state the eligibility criteria for participants and the settings and locations where the data were collected?
Interventions	Does the paper give precise details of the intervention(s) and the control intervention(s) and how and when they were administered?
Outcomes	Have the primary and secondary outcome measures been clearly defined? When applicable, have the methods used to enhance the quality of measurements (e.g. multiple observations, training of assessors) been set out?
Sample size	How was sample size determined? When applicable, were any interim analyses and/or rules for stopping the study early explained and justified?
Blinding (masking)	Does the paper state whether or not participants, those administering the interventions and those assessing the outcomes were blinded to group assignment? How was the success of blinding assessed?
Statistical methods	Were the statistical methods used to compare groups for primary and secondary outcome(s) and any subgroup analyses, appropriate?
Details of randomisation	
Sequence generation	Was the method used to generate the random allocation sequence, including details of any restrictions (e.g., blocking, stratification), clearly described?
Allocation concealment	Was the method used to implement the random allocation sequence (e.g., numbered containers or central telephone), stated, and was it made clear whether the sequence was concealed until interventions were assigned?
Implementation	Does the paper say who generated the allocation sequence, who enrolled participants and who assigned participants to their groups?

(continued overleaf)

Table 6.1 (*continued*)

Results	
Flow diagram	Is a clear diagram included showing the flow of participants through the trial? This should report, for each group, the numbers of participants randomly assigned, receiving intended treatment, completing the study protocol and analysed for the primary outcome.
Protocol deviations	Are all deviations from the original study protocol explained and justified?
Recruitment dates	Have the authors given the date range during which participants were recruited to the study?
Baseline data	Are the baseline demographic and clinical characteristics of each group described?
Numbers analysed	Is the number of participants (denominator) in each group included in each analysis, and is the analysis by 'intention-to-treat'?
Outcomes and estimation	For each primary and secondary outcome, is there a summary of results for each group, and the estimated effect size and its precision (e.g., 95% confidence interval)?
Ancillary analyses	Are all additional analyses described and justified, including subgroup analyses, both pre-specified and exploratory?
Adverse events	Have the authors reported and discussed all important adverse events?
Discussion	
Interpretation	Is the interpretation of the results justified, taking into account study hypotheses, sources of potential bias or imprecision and the dangers of multiple comparisons?
Generalisability	Have the authors made defensible estimate of the generalisability (external validity) of the trial findings?

Otherwise, the drug industry (or anyone else with a vested interest) could withhold publication of any trial that did not support their own belief in the efficacy and/or cost-effectiveness of a particular product. Goldacre [9] covers the topic of compulsory trial registration at inception (and the reluctance of some drug companies to comply with it) in his book.

Getting worthwhile evidence out of a pharmaceutical representative

Any doctor who has ever given an audience to a 'rep' who is selling a non-steroidal anti-inflammatory drug will recognise the gastric erosion example.

The question to ask him or her is not 'what is the incidence of gastric erosion on your drug?', but 'what is the incidence of potentially life-threatening gastric bleeding?'. Other questions to ask 'drug reps', based on an early article in the *Drug and Therapeutics Bulletin* [21], are listed here. For more sophisticated advice on how to debunk sponsored clinical trial reports that attempt to blind you with statistics, see Montori and colleagues' helpful Users' Guide [22] and (more tangentially but worth noting) Goldacre's blockbuster on the corporate tricks of 'big pharma' [9].

1. See representatives only by appointment. Choose to see only those whose product interests you and confine the interview to that product.
2. Take charge of the interview. Do not hear out a rehearsed sales routine but ask directly for the information.
3. Request independent published evidence from reputable peer-reviewed journals.
4. Do not look at promotional brochures, which often contain unpublished material, misleading graphs and selective quotations.
5. Ignore anecdotal 'evidence' such as the fact that a medical celebrity is prescribing the product.
6. Using the 'STEP' acronym, ask for evidence in four specific areas:
   - safety – that is, likelihood of long-term or serious side effects caused by the drug (remember that rare but serious adverse reactions to new drugs may be poorly documented);
   - tolerability, which is best measured by comparing the pooled withdrawal rates between the drug and its most significant competitor;
   - efficacy, of which the most relevant dimension is how the product compares with your current favourite; and
   - price, which should take into account indirect as well as direct costs (see section 'Ten questions to ask about an economic analysis').
7. Evaluate the evidence stringently, paying particular attention to the power (sample size) and methodological quality of clinical trials and the use of surrogate endpoints. Apply the CONSORT checklist (Table 6.1). Do not accept theoretical arguments in the drug's favour (e.g. 'longer half-life') without direct evidence that this translates into clinical benefit.
8. Do not accept the newness of a product as an argument for changing to it. Indeed, there are good scientific arguments for doing the opposite.
9. Decline to try the product via starter packs or by participating in small-scale, uncontrolled 'research' studies.
10. Record in writing the content of the interview and return to these notes if the rep requests another audience.

References

1 Godlee F. Doctors and the drug industry. BMJ 2008; 336 doi: http://dx.doi.org/10.1136/bmj.39444.472708.47.

2 Hollon MF. Direct-to-consumer advertising. JAMA: The Journal of the American Medical Association 2005;**293**(16):2030–3.

3 Liang BA, Mackey T. Direct-to-consumer advertising with interactive internet media global regulation and public health issues. JAMA: The Journal of the American Medical Association 2011;**305**(8):824–5.

4 Kaphingst KA, Dejong W, Rudd RE, et al. *A content analysis of direct-to-consumer television prescription drug advertisements. Journal of Health Communication: International Perspectives.* 2004;9(6):515–528.

5 Brody H. The company we keep: why physicians should refuse to see pharmaceutical representatives. The Annals of Family Medicine 2005;**3**(1):82–5.

6 O'brien M, Rogers S, Jamtvedt G, et al. Educational outreach visits: effects on professional practice and health care outcomes. Cochrane Database of Systematic Reviews (Online) 2007;4(4):1–6.

7 Kravitz RL, Epstein RM, Feldman MD, et al. Influence of patients' requests for direct-to-consumer advertised antidepressants. JAMA: The Journal of the American Medical Association 2005;**293**(16):1995–2002.

8 Sackett DL, Haynes RB, Tugwell P. *Clinical epidemiology: a basic science for clinical medicine.* Boston, USA: Little, Brown and Company, 1985.

9 Goldacre B. *Bad pharma: how drug companies mislead doctors and harm patients.* London, Fourth Estate: Random House Digital Inc., 2013.

10 Rajagopal S. The placebo effect. Psychiatric Bulletin 2006;**30**(5):185–8.

11 Price DD, Finniss DG, Benedetti F. A comprehensive review of the placebo effect: recent advances and current thought. Annual Review of Psychology 2008; **59**:565–90.

12 Gøtzsche PC, Liberati A, Torri V, et al. Beware of surrogate outcome measures. International Journal of Technology Assessment in Health Care 1996;**12** (02):238–46.

13 Connolly SJ. Use and misuse of surrogate outcomes in arrhythmia trials. Circulation 2006;**113**(6):764–6.

14 Guermazi A, Hayashi D, Roemer FW, et al. Osteoarthritis: a review of strengths and weaknesses of different imaging options. Rheumatic Diseases Clinics of North America 2013;**39**(3):567–91.

15 Messerli FH, Staessen JA, Zannad F. Of fads, fashion, surrogate endpoints and dual RAS blockade. European Heart Journal 2010;**31**(18):2205–8.

16 Harel Z, Gilbert C, Wald R, et al. The effect of combination treatment with aliskiren and blockers of the renin–angiotensin system on hyperkalaemia and acute kidney injury: systematic review and meta-analysis. BMJ: British Medical Journal 2012;**344**:e42.

17 Bero L. Industry sponsorship and research outcome: a Cochrane review. JAMA Internal Medicine 2013;**173**(7):580–1.

18 Schulz KF, Altman DG, Moher D. CONSORT 2010 statement: updated guidelines for reporting parallel group randomized trials. Annals of Internal Medicine 2010;**152**(11):726–32.

19 Turner L, Shamseer L, Altman DG, et al. Does use of the CONSORT Statement impact the completeness of reporting of randomised controlled trials published in medical journals? A Cochrane review. Systematic Reviews 2012;**1**:60.

20 Chalmers I, Glasziou P, Godlee F. All trials must be registered and the results published. BMJ: British Medical Journal 2013;**346**(7890):f105.

21 Herxheimer A. Getting good value from drug reps. Drug and Therapeutics Bulletin 1983;**21**:13–5.

22 Montori VM, Jaeschke R, Schünemann HJ, et al. Users' guide to detecting misleading claims in clinical research reports. BMJ: British Medical Journal 2004;**329**(7474):1093.

Chapter 7 **Papers that report trials of complex interventions**

Complex interventions

In section 'What information to expect in a paper describing a randomised controlled trial: the CONSORT statement', I defined a simple intervention (such as a drug) as one that is well demarcated (i.e. it is easy to say what the intervention comprises) and lends itself to an 'intervention on' versus 'intervention off' research design. A complex intervention is one that is not well demarcated (i.e. it is hard to say precisely what the intervention *is*) and which poses implementation challenges for researchers. Complex interventions generally involve multiple interacting components and may operate at more than one level (e.g. both individual and organisational). They include the following.

- Advice or education for patients
- Education or training for health care staff
- Interventions that seek active and ongoing input from the participant (e.g. physical activity, dietary interventions, lay support groups or psychological therapy delivered either face to face or via the Internet)
- Organisational interventions intended to increase the uptake of evidence-based practice (e.g. audit and feedback), which are discussed in more detail in Chapter 15.

Professor Penny Hawe and her colleagues [1] have argued that a complex intervention can be thought of as a 'theoretical core' (the components that make it what it is, which researchers must therefore implement faithfully) and additional non-core features that may (indeed, should) be adapted flexibly to local needs or circumstances. For example, if the intervention is providing feedback to doctors on how closely their practice aligns with an evidence-based hypertension guideline, the *core* of the intervention might be

How to Read a Paper: The Basics of Evidence-Based Medicine, Fifth Edition. Trisha Greenhalgh.
© 2014 John Wiley & Sons, Ltd. Published 2014 by John Wiley & Sons, Ltd.

information on what proportion of patients in a given time period achieved the guideline's recommended blood pressure level. The non-core elements might include how the information is given (orally, by letter and by email), whether the feedback is given as numbers or as a diagram or pie chart, whether it is given confidentially or in a group-learning situation, and so on.

Complex interventions generally need to go through a development phase so that the different components can be optimised before being tested in a full-scale randomised controlled trial. Typically, there is an initial *development* phase of qualitative interviews or observations, and perhaps a small survey to find out what people would find acceptable, which feed into the design the intervention. This is followed by a small-scale *pilot trial* (effectively a 'dress rehearsal' for a full-scale trial, in which a small number of participants are randomised to see what practical and operational issues come up), and finally the full, definitive trial [2].

Here's an example. One of my PhD students wanted to study the impact of yoga classes on the control of diabetes. She initially spent some time interviewing both people with diabetes and yoga teachers who worked with clients who had diabetes. She designed a small questionnaire to ask people with diabetes if they were interested in yoga, and found that some but not all were. All this was part of her *development phase*. The previous research literature on the therapeutic use of yoga gave her some guidance on core elements of the intervention – for example, there appeared to be good theoretical reasons why the focus should be on relaxation-type exercises rather than the more physically demanding strength or flexibility postures.

My student's initial interviews and questionnaires gave her a great deal of useful information, which she used to design the non-core elements of the yoga intervention. She knew, for example, that her potential participants were reluctant to travel very far from home, that they did not want to attend more than twice a week, that the subgroup most keen to try yoga were the recently retired (age 60–69), and that many potential participants described themselves as 'not very bendy' and were anxious not to overstretch themselves. All this information helped her design the detail of the intervention – such as who would do what, where, how often, with whom, for how long and using what materials or instruments.

To our disappointment, when we tested the carefully designed complex intervention in a randomised controlled trial, it had no impact whatsoever on diabetes control compared to waiting list controls [3]. In the discussion section of the paper reporting the findings of the yoga trial, we offered two alternative interpretations. The first interpretation was that, contrary to what previous non-randomised studies found, yoga has no effect on diabetes control. The second interpretation was that yoga may have an impact but despite our efforts in the development phase, the complex intervention was *inadequately optimised*. For example, many people found it hard to get to the group, and several people in each class did not do the exercises because they found them 'too difficult'. Furthermore, whilst the yoga teachers put a great deal of effort into the twice-weekly classes and they gave people a tape and a yoga mat to take home, they did not emphasise to participants that they should practise their exercises every day. As we discovered, hardly any of the participants did any exercises at home.

To *optimise* yoga as a complex intervention in diabetes, therefore, we might consider measures such as (i) getting a doctor or nurse to 'prescribe' it, so that the patient is more motivated to attend every class; (ii) working with the yoga teachers to design special exercises for older, under-confident people who cannot follow standard yoga exercises and (iii) stipulating more precisely what is expected as 'homework'.

This example shows that when a trial of a complex intervention produces negative results, this does not necessarily prove that all adaptations of this intervention will be ineffective in all settings. Rather, it tends to prompt the researchers to go back to the drawing board and ask how the intervention can be further refined and adapted to make it more likely to work. Note that because our yoga intervention needs more work, we did not go on directly to the full-scale randomised controlled trial but have returned to the development phase to try to refine the intervention.

Ten questions to ask about a paper describing a complex intervention

In 2008, the Medical Research Council produced updated guidance for evaluating complex interventions, and these were summarised in the *British Medical Journal* [2]. The questions given later, about how to appraise a paper describing a complex intervention, are based on this guidance.

Question One: What is the problem for which this complex intervention is seen as a possible solution?

It is all too easy to base a complex intervention study on a series of unquestioned assumptions. Teenagers drink too much alcohol and have too much unprotected sex, so surely educational programmes are needed to tell them about the dangers of this behaviour? This does not follow, of course! The problem may be teenage drinking or sexual risk-taking, but the underlying cause of that problem may not be ignorance but (for example) peer pressure and messages from the media. By considering precisely what the problem is, you will be able to look critically at whether the intervention has been (explicitly or inadvertently) designed around an appropriate theory of action (see Question Four).

Question Two: What was done in the developmental phase of the research to inform the design of the complex intervention?

There are no fixed rules about what should be done in a developmental phase, but the authors should state clearly what they did and justify it. If the developmental phase included qualitative research (this is usually the case), see Chapter 12 for detailed guidance on how to appraise such papers. If a questionnaire was used, see Chapter 14. When you have appraised the empirical work using checklists appropriate to the study design(s), consider how these findings were used to inform the design of the intervention. One aspect of the development phase will be to identify a target population and perhaps divide this into sub-populations (e.g. by age, gender, ethnicity, educational level or disease status), each of which might require the intervention to be tailored in a particular way.

Question Three: What were the core and non-core components of the intervention?

To put this question another way, (i) what are the things that should be standardised so they remain the same wherever the intervention is implemented, and (ii) what are the things that should be adapted to context and setting? The authors should state clearly which aspects of the intervention should be standardised and which should be adapted to local contingencies and priorities. An under-standardised complex intervention may lead to a paucity of generalisable findings; an over-standardised one may be unworkable in some settings and hence, overall, an under-estimate of the potential effectiveness of the core elements. The decision as to what is 'core' and what is 'non-core' should be made on the basis of the findings of the developmental phase.

Don't forget to unpack the control intervention in just as much detail as you unpack the experimental one. If the control was 'nothing' (or waiting list), describe what the participants in the control arm of the trial will *not* be receiving compared to those in the intervention arm. More likely, the control group will receive a package that includes (for example) an initial assessment, some review visits, some basic advice and perhaps a leaflet or helpline number.

Defining what the control group are offered will be particularly important if the trial addresses a controversial and expensive new care package. In a recent trial of telehealth known as the *Whole Systems Demonstrator*, the findings were interpreted by some commentators as showing that telehealth installed in people's homes leads to significantly lower use of hospital services and improved survival rates (albeit at high cost per case) [4]. However, the intervention group actually received a combination of two interventions: the telehealth equipment *and* regular phone calls from a nurse. The control group received no telehealth equipment – but no phone calls from the nurse either. Perhaps it was the human contact, not the technology, that made the difference. Frustratingly, we cannot know. In my view, the study design was flawed since it does not tell us whether telehealth 'works' or not!

Question Four: What was the theoretical mechanism of action of the intervention?

The authors of a study on a complex intervention should state explicitly how the intervention is intended to work, and that includes a statement of how the different components fit together. This statement is likely to change as the results of the developmental phase are analysed and incorporated into the refinement of the intervention.

It is not always obvious why an intervention works (or why it fails to work), especially if it involves multiple components aimed at different levels (e.g. individual, family and organisation). A few years ago, I reviewed the qualitative sections of research trials on school-based feeding programmes for disadvantaged children [5]. In 19 studies, all of which had tested this complex intervention in a randomised controlled trial (see the linked Cochrane review and meta-analysis [6]), I found a total of six different mechanisms by this intervention may have improved nutritional status, school performance or both: long-term correction of nutritional deficiencies; short-term relief of hunger; the children felt valued and looked after; reduced absenteeism; improved school diet inspired improved home diet and improved literacy in one generation improved earning power and hence reduced the risk of poverty in the next generation.

When critically appraising a paper on a complex intervention, you will need to make a judgement on whether the mechanisms offered by the authors are adequate. Common sense is a good place to start here, as is discussion among a group of experienced clinicians and service users. You may have to deduce the mechanism of action indirectly if the authors did not state it explicitly. In section 'Evaluating systematic reviews', I describe a review by Grol and Grimshaw [7], which showed that only 27% of studies of implementing evidence included an explicit theory of change.

Question Five: What outcome measures were used, and were these sensible?

With a complex intervention, a single outcome measure may not reflect all the important effects that the intervention may have. While a trial of a drug against placebo in diabetes would usually have a single primary outcome measure (typically the HbA1c blood test) and perhaps a handful of secondary outcome measures (body mass index, overall cardiovascular risk and quality of life), a trial of an educational intervention may have multiple outcomes, all of which are important in different ways. In addition to markers of diabetic control, cardiovascular risk and quality of life, it would be important to know whether staff found the educational intervention acceptable and practicable to administer, whether people showed up to the sessions, whether the participants' knowledge changed, whether they changed their self-care behaviour, whether the organisation became more patient-centred, whether calls to a helpline increased or decreased, and so on.

When you have answered questions one to five, you should be able to express a summary so far in terms of population, intervention, comparison and outcome – although this is likely to be less succinct than an equivalent summary for a simple intervention.

Question Six: What were the findings?

This is, on the surface, a simple question. But note from Question Five that a complex intervention may have significant impact on one set of outcome measures but no significant impact on other measures. Findings such as these need careful interpretation. Trials of self-management interventions (in which people with chronic illness are taught to manage their condition by altering their lifestyle and titrating their medication against symptoms or home-based tests of disease status) are widely considered to be effective. But, in fact, such programmes rarely change the underlying course of the disease or make people live longer – they just make people feel more confident in managing their illness [8, 9]! Feeling better about one's chronic illness may be an important outcome in its own right, but we need to be very precise about what complex interventions achieve – and what they don't achieve – when assessing the findings of trials.

Question Seven: What process evaluation was done – and what were the key findings of this?

A process evaluation is a (mostly) qualitative study carried out in parallel with a randomised controlled trial, which collects information on the practical challenges faced by front-line staff trying to implement the intervention [10]. In the study of yoga in diabetes, for example, researchers (one of whom was a medical student doing a BSc project) sat in on the yoga classes, interviewed patients and staff, collected the minutes of planning meetings and generally asked the question 'How's it going?'. One key finding from this was the inappropriateness of some of the venues. Only by actually being there when the yoga class was happening could we have discovered that it's impossible to relax and meditate in a public leisure centre with regular announcements over a very loud Intercom! More generally, process evaluations will capture the views of participants and staff about how to refine the intervention and/or why it may not be working as planned.

Question Eight: If the findings were negative, to what extent can this be explained by implementation failure and/or inadequate optimisation of the intervention?

This question follows on from the process evaluation. In my review of school-based feeding programmes (see Question Four), many studies had negative results, and on reading the various papers, my team came up with a number of explanations why school-based feeding might *not* improve either growth or school performance [5]. For example, the food offered may not have been consumed, or it provided too little of the key nutrients; the food consumed may have had low bioavailability in undernourished children (e.g. it was not absorbed because their intestines were oedematous); there may have been a compensatory reduction in food intake outside school (e.g. the evening meal was given to another family member if the child was known to have been fed at school); supplementation may have occurred too late in the child's development; or the programme may not have been implemented as planned (e.g. in one study, some of the control group were given food supplements because front-line staff felt, probably rightly, that it was unethical to give food to half the hungry children in a class but not the other half).

Question Nine: If the findings varied across different subgroups, to what extent have the authors explained this by refining their theory of change?

Did the intervention improve the outcomes in women but not in men? In educated middle-class people but not in uneducated or working-class people? In primary care settings but not in secondary care? Or in Manchester but not in Delhi? If so, ask why. This 'why' question is another judgement call – because it's a matter of interpreting findings in context, it can't be answered by applying a technical algorithm or checklist. Look in the discussion section of the paper and you should find the authors' explanation of why subgroup X benefited but subgroup Y didn't. They should also have offered a refinement of their theory of change that takes account of these differences. For example, the studies of school-feeding programmes showed (overall) statistically greater benefit in younger children, which led the authors of these studies to suggest that there is a critical window of development after which even nutritionally rich supplements have limited the impact on growth or performance [5, 6]. To highlight another area of interest of mine, I predict that one of the major growth areas in secondary research over the next few years will be unpacking what works for whom in education and support for self-management in different chronic conditions.

Question Ten: What further research do the authors believe is needed, and is this justified?

As you will know if you have read this chapter up to this point, complex interventions are multifaceted, nuanced and impact on multiple different outcomes. Authors who present studies of such interventions have a responsibility to tell us how their study has shaped the overall research field. They should not conclude merely that 'more research is needed' (an inevitable follow-on from any scientific study) but they should indicate *where* research efforts might best be focused. Indeed, one of the most useful conclusions might be a statement of the areas in which further research is *not* needed! The authors should state, for example, whether the next stage should be new qualitative research, a new and bigger trial or even further analysis of data already gathered.

References

1 Hawe P, Shiell A, Riley T. Complex interventions: how "out of control" can a randomised controlled trial be? BMJ: British Medical Journal 2004;**328**(7455):1561–3.

2 Craig P, Dieppe P, Macintyre S, et al. Developing and evaluating complex interventions: the new Medical Research Council guidance. BMJ: British Medical Journal 2008;**337**:a1655.

3 Skoro-Kondza L, Tai SS, Gadelrab R, et al. Community based yoga classes for type 2 diabetes: an exploratory randomised controlled trial. BMC Health Services Research 2009;**9**(1):33.

4 Steventon A, Bardsley M, Billings J, et al. Effect of telehealth on use of secondary care and mortality: findings from the Whole System Demonstrator cluster randomised trial. BMJ: British Medical Journal 2012;**344**:e3874 doi: 10.1136/bmj.e3874.

5 Greenhalgh T, Kristjansson E, Robinson V. Realist review to understand the efficacy of school feeding programmes. BMJ: British Medical Journal 2007;**335**(7625):858–61 doi: 10.1136/bmj.39359.525174.AD.

6 Kristjansson EA, Robinson V, Petticrew M, et al. School feeding for improving the physical and psychosocial health of disadvantaged elementary school children. Cochrane Database of Systematic Reviews (Online) 2007;(1):CD004676 doi: 10.1002/14651858.CD004676.pub2.

7 Grol R, Grimshaw J. From best evidence to best practice: effective implementation of change in patients' care. The Lancet 2003;**362**(9391):1225–30.

8 Foster G, Taylor S, Eldridge S, et al. Self-management education programmes by lay leaders for people with chronic conditions. Cochrane Database of Systematic Reviews (Online) 2007;4(4):1–78.

9 Nolte S, Osborne RH: A systematic review of outcomes of chronic disease self-management interventions. Quality of life research 2013, 22:1805–1816.

10 Lewin S, Glenton C, Oxman AD. Use of qualitative methods alongside randomised controlled trials of complex healthcare interventions: methodological study. BMJ: British Medical Journal 2009;339:b3496.

Chapter 8 **Papers that report diagnostic or screening tests**

Ten men in the dock

If you are new to the concept of validating diagnostic tests, and if algebraic explanations ('let's call this value x … ') leave you cold, the following example may help you. Ten men (for the gender equality purists, assume that 'men' means 'men or women') are awaiting trial for murder. Only three of them actually committed a murder; the other seven are innocent of any crime. A jury hears each case, and finds six of the men guilty of murder. Two of the convicted are true murderers. Four men are wrongly imprisoned. One murderer walks free.

This information can be expressed in what is known as a *two-by-two table* (Figure 8.1). Note that the 'truth' (i.e. whether or not each man *really* committed a murder) is expressed along the horizontal title row, whereas the jury's verdict (which may or may not reflect the truth) is expressed down the vertical title row.

You should be able to see that these figures, if they are typical, reflect a number of features of this particular jury.

(a) This jury correctly identifies two in every three true murderers.

(b) It correctly acquits three out of every seven innocent people.

(c) If this jury has found a person guilty, there is still only a one in three chance that the person is actually a murderer.

(d) If this jury found a person innocent, he has a three in four chance of actually being innocent.

(e) In 5 cases out of every 10, the jury gets the verdict right.

These five features constitute, respectively, the sensitivity, specificity, positive predictive value, negative predictive value and accuracy of this jury's performance. The rest of this chapter considers these five features applied to diagnostic (or screening) tests when compared with a 'true' diagnosis or gold

How to Read a Paper: The Basics of Evidence-Based Medicine, Fifth Edition. Trisha Greenhalgh.
© 2014 John Wiley & Sons, Ltd. Published 2014 by John Wiley & Sons, Ltd.

		True criminal status	
		Murderer	Not murderer
Jury verdict	"Guilty"	Rightly convicted **2 men**	Wrongly convicted **4 men**
	"Innocent"	**1 men** Wrongly acquitted	**3 men** Rightly acquitted

Figure 8.1 2 × 2 table showing outcome of trial for 10 men accused of murder.

standard. Section 'Likelihood ratios' also introduces a sixth, slightly more complicated (but very useful), feature of a diagnostic test – the likelihood ratio. (After you have read the rest of this chapter, look back at this section. You should, by then, be able to work out that the likelihood ratio of a positive jury verdict in the above-mentioned example is 1.17, and that of a negative one 0.78. If you can't, don't worry – many eminent clinicians have no idea what a likelihood ratio is.)

Validating diagnostic tests against a gold standard

Our window cleaner once told me that he had been feeling thirsty recently and had asked his general practitioner (GP) to be tested for diabetes, which runs in his family. The nurse in his GP's surgery had asked him to produce a urine specimen and dipped a special stick in it. The stick stayed green, which meant, apparently, that there was no sugar (glucose) in his urine. This, the nurse had said, meant that he did not have diabetes.

I had trouble explaining to the window cleaner that the test result did not necessarily mean this at all, any more than a guilty verdict *necessarily* makes someone a murderer. The definition of diabetes, according to the World Health Organisation (WHO), is a blood glucose level above 7 mmol/l in the fasting state, or above 11.1 mmol/l 2 h after a 100 g oral glucose load (the much-dreaded 'glucose tolerance test', where the participant has to glug down every last drop of a sickly glucose drink and wait 2 h for a blood test) [1]. These values must be achieved on two separate occasions if the person has no symptoms, but on only one occasion if they have typical symptoms of diabetes (thirst, passing large amounts of urine, etc.).

These stringent criteria can be termed the *gold standard* for diagnosing diabetes. In other words, if you fulfil the WHO criteria you can call yourself diabetic, and if you don't, you can't (although note that official definitions of what is and isn't a disease change regularly – and indeed, every time I produce a new edition of this book I have to see whether the ones I have cited have changed in the light of further evidence). The same cannot be said for dipping a stick into a random urine specimen. For one thing, you might be a true diabetic but have a high renal threshold – that is, your kidneys conserve glucose much better than most people's, so your blood glucose level would have to be much higher than most people's for any glucose to appear in your urine. Alternatively, you may be an otherwise normal individual with a *low* renal threshold, so glucose leaks into your urine even when there isn't any excess in your blood. In fact, as anyone with diabetes will tell you, diabetes is very often associated with a negative test for urine glucose.

There are, however, many advantages in using a urine dipstick rather than the full-blown glucose tolerance test to 'screen' people for diabetes. The test is inexpensive, convenient, easy to perform and interpret, acceptable to patients and gives an instant, yes/no result. In real life, people like my window cleaner may decline to take an oral glucose tolerance test – especially if they are self-employed and asked to miss a day's work for the test. Even if he was prepared to go ahead with it, his GP might decide (rightly or wrongly) that the window cleaner's symptoms did not merit the expense of this relatively sophisticated investigation. I hope you can see that even though the urine test cannot say for sure if someone is diabetic, it has something of a practical edge over the gold standard. That, of course, is why people use it!

In order to assess objectively just how useful the urine glucose test for diabetes is, we would need to select a sample of people (say, 100) and do two tests on each of them: the urine test (screening test), and a standard glucose tolerance test (gold standard). We could then see, for each person, whether the result of the screening test matched the gold standard. Such an exercise is known as a *validation study*. We could express the results of the validation study in a two-by-two table (also known as a *two-by-two matrix*) as in Figure 8.2, and calculate various features of the test as in Table 8.1, just as we did for the features of the jury in section 'Complex interventions'.

If the values for the various features of a test (such as sensitivity and specificity) fell within reasonable limits, we would be able to say that the test was *valid* (see Question Seven). The validity of urine testing for glucose in diagnosing diabetes was assessed many years ago by Andersson and colleagues [2], whose data I have used in the example in Figure 8.3. In fact, the original study was performed on 3268 participants, of whom 67 either refused to produce a specimen or, for some other reason, were not adequately tested. For simplicity's sake, I have ignored these irregularities and expressed the results in terms of a denominator (total number tested) of 1000 participants.

		Result of gold standard test	
		Disease positive *a + c*	Disease negative *b + d*
Result of screening test	Test positive *a + b*	True positive *a*	False positive *b*
	c + d Test negative	*c* False negative	*d* True negative

Figure 8.2 2 × 2 table notation for expressing the results of a validation study for a diagnostic or screening test.

In actual fact, these data came from an epidemiological survey to detect the prevalence of diabetes in a population; the validation of urine testing was a side issue to the main study. If the validation had been the main aim of the study, the participants selected would have included far more diabetic individuals, as Question Two in will show [2]. If you look up the original paper, you will also find that the gold standard for diagnosing true diabetes was not the oral glucose tolerance test but a more unconventional series of observations. Nevertheless, the example serves its purpose, as it provides us with some figures to put through the equations listed in the last column of Table 8.1. We can calculate the important features of the urine test for diabetes as follows:

(a) sensitivity $= a/(a + c) = 6/27 = 22.2\%$;
(b) specificity $= d/(b + d) = 966/973 = 99.3\%$;
(c) positive predictive value $= a/(a + b) = 6/13 = 46.2\%$;
(d) negative predictive value $= d/(c + d) = 966/987 = 97.9\%$;
(e) accuracy $= (a + d)/(a + b + c + d) = 972/1000 = 97.2\%$;
(f) likelihood ratio of a positive test $=$ sensitivity$/(1 - $specificity$)$
    $= 22.2/0.7 = 32$;
(g) likelihood ratio of a negative test $= (1 - $sensitivity$)/$specificity
    $= 77.8/99.3 = 0.78$.

From these features, you can probably see why I did not share the window cleaner's assurance that he did not have diabetes. A positive urine glucose test is only 22% sensitive, which means that the test misses nearly four-fifths of people who really do have diabetes. In the presence of classical symptoms and a family history, the window cleaner's baseline odds (pre-test likelihood) of having the condition are pretty high, and they are only reduced to about

Table 8.1 Features of a diagnostic test, which can be calculated by comparing it with a gold standard in a validation study

Feature of the test	Alternative name	Question that the feature addresses	Formula (see Figure 8.1)
Sensitivity	True positive rate (*Positive in Disease*)	How good is this test at picking up people who have the condition?	$a/a + c$
Specificity	True negative rate (*Negative in Health*)	How good is this test at correctly excluding people without the condition?	$d/b + d$
Positive predictive value (PPV)	Post-test probability of a positive test	If a person tests positive, what is the probability that she or he has the condition?	$a/a + b$
Negative predictive value (NPV)	Indicates the post-test probability of a negative test[a]	If a person tests negative, what is the probability that she or he does not have the condition?	$d/c + d$
Accuracy	–	What proportion of all tests have given the correct result (i.e. true positives and true negatives as a proportion of all results)?	$a + d/a + b + c + d$
Likelihood ratio of a positive test	–	How much more likely is positive test to be found in a person with, as opposed to without, the condition?	Sensitivity/(1 − specificity)

[a]The post-test probability of a negative test is (1 − NPV).

		Result of gold standard glucose tolerance test	
		Diabetes positive 27 people	Diabetes negative 973 people
Result of urine test for glucose	Glucose present 13 people	True positive 6	False positive 7
	987 people Glucose absent	21 False negative	966 True negative

Figure 8.3 2 × 2 table showing results of a validation study of urine glucose testing for diabetes against the gold standard of glucose tolerance test (based on Andersson et al. [2]).

four-fifths of this (the negative likelihood ratio, 0.78; see section 'Likelihood ratios') after a single negative urine test. In view of his symptoms, this man clearly needs to undergo a more definitive test for diabetes [3]. Note that as the definitions in Table 8.1 show, if the test had been positive the window cleaner would have good reason to be concerned, because even though the test is not very *sensitive* (i.e. it is not good at picking up people with the disease), it is pretty *specific* (i.e. it *is* good at excluding people without the disease).

Despite the findings of these studies from almost 20 years ago, urine testing to 'exclude diabetes' is still shockingly common in some settings. But the academic argument has long shifted to the question of whether the HbA1c blood test is sufficiently sensitive and specific to serve as a screening test for diabetes [4, 5]. The arguments have become far more complex as epidemiologists have weighed in with evidence on early (subclinical) microvascular damage, but the essential principles of the 2 × 2 matrix and the questions about false positives and false negatives still apply. In short, the test performs very well – but it does require a blood test and the costs are not insignificant.

Students often get mixed up about the sensitivity/specificity dimension of a test and the positive/negative predictive value dimension. As a rule of thumb, the sensitivity or specificity tells you about the *test in general*, whereas the predictive value tells you about *what a particular test result means for the patient in front of you*. Hence, sensitivity and specificity are generally used more by epidemiologists and public health specialists whose day-to-day work involves making decisions about *populations*.

A screening mammogram (breast X-ray) might have an 80% sensitivity and a 90% specificity for detecting breast cancer, which means that the test will pick up 80% of cancers and exclude 90% of women without cancer. But imagine you were a GP or practice nurse and a patient comes to see you for the result of her mammogram. The question she will want answered is (if the test has come back positive), 'What is the chance that I've got cancer?' or (if it has come back negative) 'What is the chance that I can now forget about the possibility of cancer?' Many patients (and far too many health professionals) assume that the negative predictive value of a test is 100% – that is, if the test is 'normal' or 'clear' they think there is no chance of the disease being present – and you only need to read the confessional stories in women's magazines ('I was told I had cancer but tests later proved the doctors wrong') to find examples of women who have assumed that the positive predictive value of a test is 100%.

Ten questions to ask about a paper that claims to validate a diagnostic or screening test

In preparing these tips, I have drawn on three main published sources: the Users' Guides to the Medical Literature [6, 7]; a more recent article by some of the same authors [8] and Mant's [9] simple and pragmatic guidelines for 'testing a test'. Like many of the checklists in this book, these are no more than pragmatic rules-of-thumb for the novice critical appraiser: for a much more comprehensive and rigorously developed set of criteria (which runs to a daunting 234 pages) known as the *QADAS* (Quality in Diagnostic and Screening tests) checklist, see a recent review by the UK Health Technology Assessment Programme [8]. Lucas and colleagues [10] have since produced a checklist that is similar but not identical to the questions listed here.

Question One: Is this test potentially relevant to my practice?

This is the 'so what?' question, which epidemiologists call the *utility* of the test. Even if this test were 100% valid, accurate and reliable, would it help me? Would it identify a treatable disorder? If so, would I use it in preference to the test I use now? Could I (or my patients or the taxpayer) afford it? Would my patients consent to it? Would it change the probabilities for competing diagnoses sufficiently for me to alter my treatment plan? If the answers to these questions are all 'no', you may be able to reject the paper without reading further than the abstract or introduction.

Question Two: Has the test been compared with a true gold standard?

You need to ask, first, whether the test has been compared with anything at all! Papers have occasionally been written (and, in the past, published) in which nothing has been done except perform the new test on a few dozen participants. This exercise may give a range of possible results for the test, but it certainly does not confirm that the 'high' results indicate that target disorder (the disease or risk state that you are interested in) is present or that the 'low' results indicate that it isn't.

Next, you should verify that the 'gold standard' test used in the survey merits the term. A good way of assessing a gold standard is to use the 'so what?' questions listed earlier. For many conditions, there is no absolute gold standard diagnostic test that will say for certain if it is present or not. Unsurprisingly, these tend to be the very conditions for which new tests are most actively sought! Hence, the authors of such papers may need to develop and justify a combination of criteria against which the new test is to be assessed. One specific point to check is that the test being validated here (or a variant of it) is not being used to contribute to the definition of the gold standard.

Question Three: Did this validation study include an appropriate spectrum of participants?

If you validated a new test for cholesterol in 100 healthy male medical students, you would not be able to say how the test would perform in women, children, older people, those with diseases that seriously raise the cholesterol level, or even those who had never been to medical school. Although few people would be naive enough to select quite such a biased sample for their validation study, it is surprisingly common for published studies to omit to define the spectrum of participants tested in terms of age, gender, symptoms and/or disease severity and specific eligibility criteria.

Defining both the range of participants and the spectrum of disease to be included is essential if the values for the different features of the test are to be worth quoting – that is, if they are to be transferable to other settings. A particular diagnostic test may, conceivably, be more sensitive in female participants than in male participants, or in younger rather than in older participants. For the same reasons, the participants on which any test is verified should include those with both mild and severe disease, treated and untreated and those with different but commonly confused conditions.

Whilst the sensitivity and specificity of a test are virtually constant whatever the prevalence of the condition, the positive and negative predictive values are crucially dependent on prevalence. This is why GPs are, often rightly, sceptical of the utility of tests developed exclusively in a secondary care population, where the severity of disease tends to be greater (see section 'Whom is the study about?'), and why a good *diagnostic* test (generally used when the patient has some symptoms suggestive of the disease in question) is not necessarily a good *screening* test (generally used in people without symptoms, who are drawn from a population with a much lower prevalence of the disease).

Question Four: Has work-up (verification) bias been avoided?

This is easy to check. It simply means, 'did everyone who got the new diagnostic test also get the gold standard, and vice versa?'. I hope you have no problem spotting the potential bias in studies where the gold standard test is only performed on people who have already tested positive for the test being validated. There are, in addition, a number of more subtle aspects of work-up or verification bias that are beyond the scope of this book but which are covered in specialist statistics textbooks [11].

Question Five: Has expectation bias been avoided?

Expectation bias occurs when pathologists and others who interpret diagnostic specimens are subconsciously influenced by the knowledge of the particular features of the case – for example, the presence of chest pain when interpreting an electrocardiogram (ECG). In the context of validating diagnostic tests against a gold standard, the question means, 'did the people who interpreted one of the tests know what result the other test had shown on each particular participant?'. As I explained in section 'Was assessment "blind"?', all assessments should be 'blind' – that is, the person interpreting the test should not be given any inkling of what the result is expected to be in any particular case.

Question Six: Was the test shown to be reproducible both within and between observers?

If the same observer performs the same test on two occasions on a participant whose characteristics have not changed, they will get different results in a proportion of cases. All tests show this feature to some extent, but a test with a reproducibility of 99% is clearly in a different league from one with a reproducibility of 50%. A number of factors that may contribute to the poor reproducibility of a diagnostic test are the technical precision of the equipment, observer variability (e.g. in comparing a colour with a reference chart), arithmetical errors and so on.

Look back again at section 'Was assessment "blind"?' to remind yourself of the problem of inter-observer agreement. Given the same result to interpret, two people will agree in only a proportion of cases, generally expressed as the Kappa score. If the test in question gives results in terms of numbers (such as the serum cholesterol level in millimole per litre), inter-observer agreement is hardly an issue. If, however, the test involves reading X-rays (such as the mammogram example in Section 'Was assessment "blind"?') or asking a person questions about their drinking habits [10], it is important to confirm that reproducibility between observers is at an acceptable level.

Question Seven: What are the features of the test as derived from this validation study?

All these standards could have been met, but the test may still be worthless because the test itself is not valid (i.e. its sensitivity, specificity and other crucial features are too low. That is clearly the case for using urine glucose to screen for diabetes; see section 'Ten questions to ask about a paper describing a complex intervention'). After all, if a test has a false-negative rate of nearly 80%, it is more likely to mislead the clinician than assist the diagnosis if the target disorder is actually present.

There are no absolutes for the validity of a screening test, because what counts as acceptable depends on the condition being screened for. Few of us would quibble about a test for colour blindness that was 95% sensitive and 80% specific, but nobody ever died of colour blindness. The Guthrie heel-prick screening test for congenital hypothyroidism, performed on all babies in the UK soon after birth, is over 99% sensitive but has a positive predictive value of only 6% (in other words, it picks up almost all babies with the condition at the expense of a high false-positive rate) [11], and rightly so. It is far more important to pick up every single baby with this treatable condition who would otherwise develop severe mental handicap than to save hundreds of parents the relatively minor stress of a repeat blood test on their baby.

Question Eight: Were confidence intervals given for sensitivity, specificity and other features of the test?

As section 'Probability and confidence' explained, a confidence interval, which can be calculated for virtually every numerical aspect of a set of results, expresses the possible range of results within which the true value will lie. Go back to the jury example in section 'Complex interventions'. If they had found just one more murderer not guilty, the sensitivity of their verdict would have gone down from 67% to 33%, and the positive predictive value of the verdict from 33% to 20%. This enormous (and quite unacceptable) sensitivity to a single case decision is because we only validated the jury's performance on 10 cases. The confidence intervals for the features of this jury are so wide that my computer programme refuses to calculate them! Remember, the larger the sample size, the narrower the confidence interval, so it is particularly important to look for confidence intervals if the paper you are reading reports a study on a relatively small sample. If you would like the formula for calculating confidence intervals for diagnostic test features, see the excellent textbook 'Statistics with Confidence' [12].

Question Nine: Has a sensible 'normal range' been derived from these results?

If the test gives non-dichotomous (continuous) results – in other words, if it gives a numerical value rather than a yes/no result – someone will have to say at what value the test result will count as abnormal. Many of us have been there with our own blood pressure reading. We want to know if our result is 'okay' or not, but the doctor insists on giving us a value such as '142/92'. If 140/90 were chosen as the cut-off for high blood pressure, we would be placed in the 'abnormal' category, even though our risk of problems from our blood pressure is very little different from that of a person with a blood pressure of 138/88. Quite sensibly, many practising doctors and nurses advise their patients, 'Your blood pressure isn't quite right, but it doesn't fall into the danger zone. Come back in three months for another check'. Nevertheless, the clinician must at some stage make the decision that *this* blood pressure needs treating with tablets but *this* one does not. When and how often to repeat a borderline test is often addressed in guidelines – you might, for example, like to look up the detailed guidance and prevailing controversies on how to measure blood pressure [13]. Defining relative and absolute danger zones for a continuous physiological or pathological variable is a complex science, which should take into account the actual likelihood of the adverse outcome that the proposed treatment aims to prevent. This process is made considerably more objective by the use of likelihood ratios (see section 'Likelihood ratios'). For an entertaining discussion on the different possible meanings of the word 'normal' in diagnostic investigations, see Sackett and colleagues' [14] textbook, p. 59.

Question Ten: Has this test been placed in the context of other potential tests in the diagnostic sequence for the condition?

In general, we treat high blood pressure on the basis of the blood pressure reading alone (although as mentioned, guidelines recommend basing management on a series of readings rather than a single value). Compare this with the sequence we use to diagnose stenosis ('hardening') of the coronary arteries. First, we select patients with a typical history of effort angina (chest pain on exercise). Next, we usually do a resting ECG, an exercise ECG, and, in some cases, a radionucleide scan of the heart to look for areas short of oxygen. Most patients only come to a coronary angiogram (the definitive investigation for coronary artery stenosis) *after* they have produced an abnormal result on these preliminary tests.

If you took 100 people off the street and sent them straight for a coronary angiogram, the test might display very different positive and negative predictive values (and even different sensitivity and specificity) than it did in the sicker population on which it was originally validated. This means that the various aspects of validity of the coronary angiogram as a diagnostic test are virtually meaningless unless these figures are expressed in terms of what they contribute to the overall diagnostic work-up.

Likelihood ratios

Question Nine described the problem of defining a normal range for a continuous variable. In such circumstances, it can be preferable to express the test result not as 'normal' or 'abnormal', but in terms of the actual chances of a patient having the target disorder if the test result reaches a particular level. Take, for example, the use of the prostate-specific antigen (PSA) test to screen for prostate cancer. Most men will have some detectable PSA in their blood (say, 0.5 ng/ml), and most of those with advanced prostate cancer will have very high levels of PSA (above about 20 ng/ml). But a PSA level of, say, 7.4 ng/ml may be found either in a perfectly normal man or in someone with early cancer. There simply is not a clean cut-off between normal and abnormal [15].

We can, however, use the results of a validation study of the PSA test against a gold standard for prostate cancer (say, a biopsy) to draw up a whole series of two-by-two tables. Each table would use a different definition of an abnormal PSA result to classify patients as 'normal' or 'abnormal'. From these tables, we could generate different likelihood ratios associated with a PSA level above each different cut-off point. Then, when faced with a PSA result in the 'grey zone', we would at least be able to say, 'this test has not proved that the patient has prostate cancer, but it has increased [or decreased] the odds of that diagnosis by a factor of x'. In fact, as I mentioned earlier, the PSA test is not a terribly good discriminator between the presence and absence of cancer, whatever cut-off value is used – in other words, there is no value for PSA that gives a particularly high likelihood ratio in cancer detection. The latest advice is to share these uncertainties with the patient and let him decide whether to have the test [16].

Although the likelihood ratio is one of the more complicated aspects of a diagnostic test to calculate, it has enormous practical value, and it is becoming the preferred way of expressing and comparing the usefulness of different tests. The likelihood ratio is a particularly helpful test for ruling a particular diagnosis in or out. For example, if a person enters my consulting room with no symptoms at all, I know (on the basis of some rather old epidemiological studies) that they have a 5% chance of having iron-deficiency anaemia, because around one person in 20 in the UK population has this condition. In the language of diagnostic tests, this means that the pre-test probability of anaemia, equivalent to the prevalence of the condition, is 0.05.

Now, if I carry out a diagnostic test for anaemia, the serum ferritin level, the result will usually make the diagnosis of anaemia either more or less likely. A moderately reduced serum ferritin level (between 18 and 45 µg/l) has a likelihood ratio of 3, so the chances of a patient with this result having iron-deficiency anaemia is generally calculated as 0.05×3 – or 0.15 (15%). This value is known as the *post-test probability of the serum ferritin test*. (Strictly speaking, likelihood ratios should be used on odds rather than on probabilities, but the simpler method shown here gives a good approximation when the pre-test probability is low. In this example, a pre-test probability of 5% is equal to a pre-test odds of 0.05/0.95 or 0.053; a positive test with a likelihood ratio of 3 gives a post-test odds of 0.158, which is equal to a post-test probability of 14%) [17].

Figure 8.4 shows a nomogram, adapted by Sackett and colleagues from an original paper by Fagan [18], for working out post-test probabilities when the pre-test probability (prevalence) and likelihood ratio for the test are known. The lines A, B and C, drawn from a pre-test probability of 25% (the prevalence of smoking amongst British adults) are, respectively, the trajectories through likelihood ratios of 15, 100 and 0.015 – three different (and all somewhat old) tests for detecting whether someone is a smoker [19]. Actually, test C detects whether the person is a *non-smoker*, as a positive result in this test leads to a post-test probability of only 0.5%.

In summary, as I said at the beginning of this chapter, you can go a long way with diagnostic tests without referring to likelihood ratios. I avoided them myself for years. But if you put aside an afternoon to get to grips with this aspect of clinical epidemiology, I predict that your time will have been well spent.

Clinical prediction rules

In the previous section, I took you through a rather heavy-going example of the PSA test, and concluded that there is no single, clear-cut value that reliably distinguishes 'normal' from 'abnormal'. This is why the recommended approach to assessing a man's risk of prostate cancer is a combination of several tests, including the overall clinical assessment and a digital rectal examination [16].

More generally, you can probably see why, in general, clinicians tend to use a combination of several different diagnostic tests (including their clinical examination, blood tests, X-rays, etc.) to build up a picture of what is wrong with the patient. Whilst any one test has a fuzzy boundary between normal and abnormal, combining them may sharpen the diagnostic focus. So, for example, a woman who presents with a breast lump tends to be offered three different tests, none of which is especially useful when used in isolation: fine needle aspiration, X-ray (mammogram) and ultrasound [20]. More recently, scholars have begun a debate as to whether computerised mammography reading increases the accuracy of this triple combination further [21].

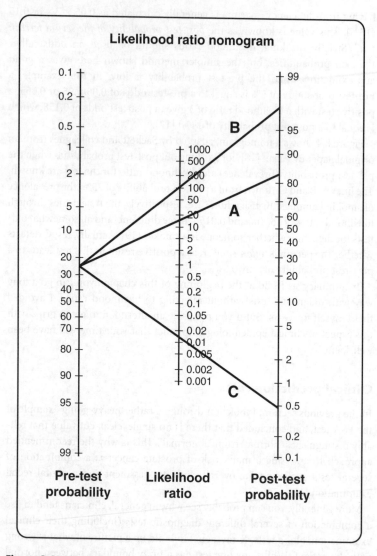

Figure 8.4 Using likelihood ratios to calculating the post-test probability of someone being a smoker.

This general principle – do several tests and combine them – is a longstanding rule of thumb in clinical practice, recently updated in a more structured form by Falk and Fahey [22]. By following large cohorts of patients with particular symptoms, and carefully recording the findings of clinical examinations and diagnostic tests in all of them, we can come up with numerical estimates of the chance of a person having (or going on to develop) disease X in the presence of symptom A, physical sign B, diagnostic test C, and so on – or any combination of these. Interest in – and research into – clinical prediction rules has been growing rapidly in recent years, partly because the growth of information technology means that very large numbers of patients can be entered onto online databases by clinicians in different centres.

As Falk and Fahey point out, there are three stages in the development of a clinical prediction rule. First, the rule must be developed by establishing the independent and combined effect of explanatory variables such as symptoms, signs, or diagnostic tests on the diagnosis. Second, these explanatory variables should be assessed in different populations. And third, there should be an impact analysis – ideally a randomised trial that measures the impact of applying the rule in a clinical setting in terms of patient outcome, clinician behaviour, resource use, and so on.

For examples of how clinical prediction rules can help us work through some of the knottiest diagnostic challenges in health care, see these papers on how to predict whether a head-injured child should be sent for a computed tomography (CT) scan [23], whether someone with early arthritis is developing rheumatoid arthritis [24], whether someone taking anticoagulants is of sufficiently low risk of stroke to be able to discontinue them [25], and which combinations of tests best predict whether an acutely ill child has anything serious wrong with him or her [26].

References

1 World Health Organization. Definition and diagnosis of diabetes mellitus and intermediate hyperglycemia: report of a WHO/IDF consultation. Geneva: World Health Organization, 2006:1–50.

2 Andersson D, Lundblad E, Svärdsudd K. A model for early diagnosis of type 2 diabetes mellitus in primary health care. Diabetic Medicine 1993;**10**(2):167–73.

3 Friderichsen B, Maunsbach M. Glycosuric tests should not be employed in population screenings for NIDDM. Journal of Public Health 1997;**19**(1):55–60.

4 Bennett C, Guo M, Dharmage S. HbA1c as a screening tool for detection of type 2 diabetes: a systematic review. Diabetic Medicine 2007;**24**(4):333–43.

5 Lu ZX, Walker KZ, O'Dea K, et al. A1C for screening and diagnosis of type 2 diabetes in routine clinical practice. Diabetes Care 2010;**33**(4):817–9.

6 Jaeschke R, Guyatt G, Sackett DL, et al. Users' guides to the medical literature: III. How to use an article about a diagnostic test. A. Are the results of the study valid? JAMA: The Journal of the American Medical Association – US Edition 1994;**271**(5):389–91.

7 Guyatt G, Bass E, Brill-Edwards P, et al. Users' guides to the medical literature: III. How to use an article about a diagnostic test. B. What are the results and will they help me in caring for my patients? JAMA: The Journal of American Medical Association 1994;**271**(9):703–7.

8 Guyatt G, Sackett D, Haynes B. Evaluating diagnostic tests. *Clinical epidemiology: how to do clinical practice research* 2006;**424**:273–322.

9 Mant D. Testing a test: three critical steps. Oxford General Practice Series 1995;**28**:183.

10 Lucas NP, Macaskill P, Irwig L, et al. The development of a quality appraisal tool for studies of diagnostic reliability (QAREL). Journal of Clinical Epidemiology 2010;**63**(8):854–61.

11 Lu Y, Dendukuri N, Schiller I, et al. A Bayesian approach to simultaneously adjusting for verification and reference standard bias in diagnostic test studies. Statistics in Medicine 2010;**29**(24):2532–43.

12 Altman DG, Machin D, Bryant TN, et al. *Statistics with confidence: confidence intervals and statistical guidelines.* Bristol: BMJ Books, 2000.

13 Appel LJ, Miller ER, Charleston J. Improving the measurement of blood pressure: is it time for regulated standards? Annals of Internal Medicine. 2011;**154**(12):838–9.

14 Sackett DL, Haynes RB, Tugwell P. *Clinical epidemiology: a basic science for clinical medicine.* Boston: Little, Brown and Company, 1985.

15 Holmström B, Johansson M, Bergh A, et al. Prostate specific antigen for early detection of prostate cancer: longitudinal study. BMJ: British Medical Journal 2009;**339**:b3537.

16 Barry M, Denberg T, Owens D, et al. Screening for prostate cancer: a guidance statement from the Clinical Guidelines Committee of the American College of Physicians. Annals of Internal Medicine 2013;**158**:761–9.

17 Guyatt GH, Patterson C, Ali M, et al. Diagnosis of iron-deficiency anemia in the elderly. The American Journal of Medicine 1990;**88**(3):205–9.

18 Fagan TJ. Letter: nomogram for Bayes theorem. The New England Journal of Medicine 1975;**293**(5):257.

19 Moore A, McQuay H, Muir Gray J. How good is that test – using the result. Bandolier. Oxford 1996;**3**(6):6–8.

20 Houssami N, Irwig L. Likelihood ratios for clinical examination, mammography, ultrasound and fine needle biopsy in women with breast problems. The Breast 1998;**7**(2):85–9.

21 Giger ML. Update on the potential of computer-aided diagnosis for breast cancer. Future Oncology 2010;**6**(1):1–4.

22 Falk G, Fahey T. Clinical prediction rules. BMJ: British Medical Journal 2009;**339**:b2899.

23 Maguire JL, Boutis K, Uleryk EM, et al. Should a head-injured child receive a head CT scan? A systematic review of clinical prediction rules. Pediatrics 2009;**124**(1):e145–54.

24 Kuriya B, Cheng CK, Chen HM, et al. Validation of a prediction rule for development of rheumatoid arthritis in patients with early undifferentiated arthritis. Annals of the Rheumatic Diseases 2009;**68**(9):1482–5.

25 Rodger MA, Kahn SR, Wells PS, et al. Identifying unprovoked thromboembolism patients at low risk for recurrence who can discontinue anticoagulant therapy. Canadian Medical Association Journal 2008;**179**(5):417–26.

26 Verbakel JY, Van den Bruel A, Thompson M, et al. How well do clinical prediction rules perform in identifying serious infections in acutely ill children across an international network of ambulatory care datasets? BMC Medicine 2013;**11**(1):10.

Chapter 9   **Papers that summarise other papers (systematic reviews and meta-analyses)**

When is a review systematic?

Remember the essays you used to write when you first started college? You would mooch round the library, browsing through the indexes of books and journals. When you came across a paragraph that looked relevant you copied it out, and if anything you found did not fit in with the theory you were proposing, you left it out. This, more or less, constitutes the *journalistic* review – an overview of primary studies that have not been identified or analysed in a systematic (i.e. standardised and objective) way. Journalists get paid according to how much they write rather than how much they read or how critically they process it, which explains why most of the 'new scientific breakthroughs' you read in your newspaper today will probably be discredited before the month is out. A common variant of the journalistic review is the invited review, written when an editor asks one of his or her friends to pen a piece, and summed up by this fabulous title: 'The invited review? Or, my field, from my standpoint, written by me using only my data and my ideas, and citing only my publications' [1]!

In contrast, a *systematic review* is an overview of primary studies which:
- contains a statement of objectives, sources and methods;
- has been conducted in a way that is explicit, transparent and reproducible (see Figure 9.1).

The most enduring and reliable systematic reviews, notably those undertaken by the Cochrane Collaboration (see section 'Specialised resources') are regularly updated to incorporate new evidence.

As my colleague Paul Knipschild observed some years ago, Nobel Prize winner Pauling [2] once published a review, based on selected referencing of the studies that supported his hypothesis, showing that vitamin C cured the common cold. A more objective analysis showed that whilst one of two did indeed suggest an effect, a true estimate based on *all* the available studies

---

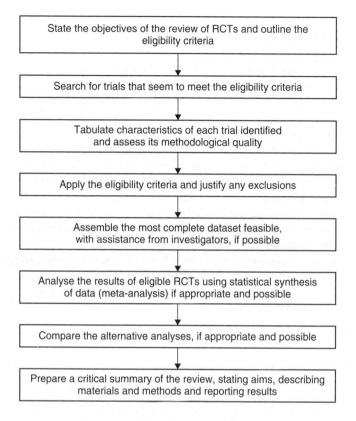

Figure 9.1 Method for a systematic review.

suggested that vitamin C had no effect at all on the course of the common cold. Pauling probably did not deliberately intend to deceive his readers, but because his enthusiasm for his espoused cause outweighed his scientific objectivity, he was unaware of the *selection bias* influencing his choice of papers. Evidence shows that if you or I were to attempt what Pauling did – that is, hunt through the medical literature for 'evidence' to support our pet theory – we would make an equally idiosyncratic and unscientific job of it [3]. Some advantages of the systematic review are given in Box 9.1.

Experts, who have been steeped in a subject for years and know what the answer 'ought' to be, were once shown to be significantly less able to produce an objective review of the literature in their subject than non-experts [4]. This would have been of little consequence if experts' opinion could be relied upon to be congruent with the results of independent systematic reviews,

Box 9.1 Advantages of systematic reviews [2]

- Explicit methods *limit bias* in identifying and rejecting studies.
- Conclusions are hence more *reliable* and *accurate*.
- Large amounts of *information* can be assimilated quickly by health care providers, researchers and policymakers.
- Delay between research discoveries and *implementation* of effective diagnostic and therapeutic strategies is reduced (see Chapter 12).
- Results of different studies can be formally compared to establish *generalisability* of findings and *consistency* (lack of heterogeneity) of results (see section 'Likelihood ratios').
- Reasons for *heterogeneity* (inconsistency in results across studies) can be identified and new hypotheses generated about particular subgroups (see section 'Likelihood ratios').
- Quantitative systematic reviews (meta-analyses) increase the *precision* of the overall result (see sections 'Were preliminary statistical questions addressed?' and 'Ten questions to ask about a paper that claims to validate a diagnostic or screening test').

but at the time they most certainly couldn't [5]. These condemning studies are still widely quoted by people who would replace all subject experts (such as cardiologists) with search-and-appraisal experts (people who specialise in finding and criticising papers on any subject). But no one in more recent years has replicated the findings – in other words, perhaps we should credit today's experts with more of a tendency to base their recommendations on a thorough assessment of the evidence! As a general rule, if you want to seek out the best objective evidence of the benefits of (say) different anticoagulants in atrial fibrillation, you should ask someone who is an expert in systematic reviews to work alongside an expert in atrial fibrillation.

To be fair to Pauling [2], he did mention a number of trials whose results seriously challenged his theory that vitamin C prevents the common cold. But he described all such trials as 'methodologically flawed'. So were many of the trials that Pauling *did* include in his analysis, but because their results were consistent with Pauling's views, he was, perhaps subconsciously, less critical of weaknesses in their design [6].

I mention this example to illustrate the point that, when undertaking a systematic review, not only must the search for relevant articles be thorough and objective but the criteria used to reject articles as 'flawed' must be explicit and independent of the results of those trials. In other words, you don't trash a trial because all other trials in this area showed something different (see section 'Explaining heterogeneity'); you trash it because, *whatever the results showed*, the trial's objectives or methods did not meet your inclusion criteria or quality standard (see section 'The science of "trashing" papers').

Evaluating systematic reviews

One of the major developments in evidence-based medicine (EBM) since I wrote the first edition of this book in 1995 has been the agreement on a standard, structured format for writing up and presenting systematic reviews. The original version of this was called the *QUORUM statement* (equivalent to the CONSORT format for reporting randomised controlled trials discussed in section 'Randomised controlled trials'). It was subsequently updated as the Preferred Reporting Items for Systematic Reviews and Meta-Analyses (PRISMA) statement [7]. Following these structured checklists makes systematic reviews and meta-analyses a whole lot easier to find your way around. Here are some questions based on the PRISMA checklist (but greatly shortened and simplified) to ask about any systematic review of quantitative evidence.

Question One: What is the important clinical question that the review addressed?

Look back to Chapter 3, in which I explained the importance of defining the question when reading a paper about a clinical trial or other form of primary research. I called this *getting your bearings* because one sure way to be confused about a paper is to fail to ascertain what it is about. The definition of a specific answerable question is, if anything, even more important (and even more frequently omitted!) when preparing an overview of primary studies. If you have ever tried to pull together the findings of a dozen or more clinical papers into an essay, editorial or summary notes for an examination, you will know that it is all too easy to meander into aspects of the topic that you never intended to cover.

The question addressed by a systematic review needs to be defined very precisely, as the reviewer must make a dichotomous (yes/no) decision as to whether each potentially relevant paper will be included or, alternatively, rejected as 'irrelevant'. The question, 'do anticoagulants prevent strokes in patients with atrial fibrillation?' sounds pretty specific, until you start looking through the list of possible studies to include. Does 'atrial fibrillation' include both rheumatic and non-rheumatic forms (which are known to be associated with very different risks of stroke), and does it include intermittent atrial fibrillation? My grandfather, for example, used to go into this arrhythmia for a few hours on the rare occasions when he drank coffee and would have counted as a 'grey case' in any trial.

Does 'stroke' include both ischaemic stroke (caused by a *blocked* blood vessel in the brain) and haemorrhagic stroke (caused by a *burst* blood vessel)? And, talking of burst blood vessels, shouldn't we be weighing the side effects of anticoagulants against their possible benefits? Does 'anticoagulant' mean the narrow sense of the term (i.e. drugs that work on the clotting cascade) such as heparin, warfarin and dabigatran, or does it also include drugs that reduce platelet stickiness, such as aspirin and clopidogrel? Finally, should the review cover trials on people who have already had a previous stroke or transient ischaemic attack (a mild stroke that gets better within 24 h), or should it be limited to trials on individuals without these major risk factors for a further stroke? The 'simple' question posed earlier is becoming unanswerable, and we must refine it in this manner.

> To assess the effectiveness and safety of warfarin-type anticoagulant therapy in secondary prevention (i.e. following a previous stroke or transient ischaemic attack) in patients with all forms of atrial fibrillation: comparison with antiplatelet therapy [8].

Question Two: Was a thorough search carried out of the appropriate database(s) and were other potentially important sources explored?

As Figure 9.1 illustrates, one of the benefits of a systematic review is that, unlike a narrative or journalistic review, the author is required to tell you where the information in it came from and how it was processed. As I explained in Chapter 2, searching the Medline database for relevant articles is a sophisticated science, and even the best Medline search will miss important papers. The reviewer who seeks a comprehensive set of primary studies must approach the other databases listed in section 'Primary studies – tackling the jungle' – and sometimes many more (e.g. in a systematic review of the diffusion of innovations in health service organisations, my colleagues and I searched a total of 15 databases, 9 of which I'd never even heard of when I started the study [9]).

In the search for trials to include in a review, the scrupulous avoidance of linguistic imperialism is a scientific as well as a political imperative. As much weight must be given, for example, to the expressions 'Eine Placebo-kontrollierte Doppel-blindstudie' and 'une étude randomisée a double insu face au placebo' as to 'a double-blind, randomised controlled trial' [6], although omission of other-language studies is not, generally, associated with biased results (it's just bad science) [10]. Furthermore, particularly where a statistical synthesis of results (meta-analysis) is contemplated, it may be necessary to write and ask the authors of the primary studies for data that were not originally included in the published review (see section 'Meta-analysis for the non-statistician').

Even when all this has been done, the systematic reviewer's search for material has hardly begun. As Knipschild and colleagues [6] showed when they searched for trials on vitamin C and cold prevention, their electronic databases only gave them 22 of their final total of 61 trials. Another 39 trials were uncovered by hand-searching the manual Index Medicus database (14 trials not identified previously), and searching the references of the trials identified in Medline (15 more trials), the references of the references (9 further trials), and the references of the references of the references (one additional trial not identified by any of the previous searches).

Do not be too hard on a reviewer, however, if he or she has not followed this counsel of perfection to the letter. After all, Knipschild and his team [6] found that only one of the trials not identified in Medline met stringent criteria for methodological quality and ultimately contributed to their systematic review of vitamin C in cold prevention. The use of more laborious search methods (such as pursuing the references of references, citation chaining writing to all the known experts in the field, and hunting out 'grey literature') (see Box 9.2 and also section 'Primary studies – tackling the jungle') may be of greater relative importance when looking at trials outside the medical mainstream. For example, in health service management, my own team showed that only around a quarter of relevant, high-quality papers were turned up by electronic searching [11].

Question Three: Was methodological quality assessed and the trials weighted accordingly?

Chapters 3 and 4 and Appendix 1 provide some checklists for assessing whether a paper should be rejected outright on methodological grounds. But given that only around 1% of clinical trials are said to be beyond

---

Box 9.2 Checklist of data sources for a systematic review

- Medline database
- Cochrane controlled clinical trials register (see 'Synthesised sources', page 17)
- Other medical and paramedical databases (see the whole of Chapter 2, page 15)
- Foreign language literature
- 'Grey literature' (theses, internal reports, non-peer-reviewed journals, pharmaceutical industry files)
- References (and references of references, etc.) listed in primary sources
- Other unpublished sources known to experts in the field (seek by personal communication)
- Raw data from published trials (seek by personal communication)

criticism methodologically, the practical question is how to ensure that a 'small but perfectly formed' study is given the weight it deserves in relation to a larger study whose methods are adequate but more open to criticism. As the PRISMA statement emphasises, the key question is the extent to which the methodological flaws are likely to have *biased* the review's findings [7].

Methodological shortcomings that invalidate the results of trials are often generic (i.e. they are independent of the subject matter of the study; see Appendix 1), but there may also be certain methodological features that distinguish between good, medium and poor quality in a particular field. Hence, one of the tasks of a systematic reviewer is to draw up a list of criteria, including both generic and particular aspects of quality, against which to judge each trial. In theory, a composite numerical score could be calculated which would reflect 'overall methodological quality'. In reality, however, care should be taken in developing such scores as there is no gold standard for the 'true' methodological quality of a trial and such composite scores may prove neither valid nor reliable in practice. If you're interested in reading more about the science of developing and applying quality criteria to studies as part of a systematic review, see the latest edition of the Cochrane Reviewers' Handbook [12].

Question Four: How sensitive are the results to the way the review has been performed?

If you don't understand what this question means, look up the tongue-in-cheek paper by Counsell and colleagues [13] some years ago in the *British Medical Journal*, which 'proved' an entirely spurious relationship between the result of shaking a dice and the outcome of an acute stroke. The authors report a series of artificial dice-rolling experiments in which red, white and green dice, respectively, represented different therapies for acute stroke.

Overall, the 'trials' showed no significant benefit from the three therapies. However, the simulation of a number of perfectly plausible events in the process of meta-analysis – such as the exclusion of several of the 'negative' trials through publication bias (see section 'Randomised controlled trials'), a subgroup analysis that excluded data on red dice therapy (because, on looking back at the results, red dice appeared to be harmful), and other, essentially arbitrary, exclusions on the grounds of 'methodological quality' – led to an apparently highly significant benefit of 'dice therapy' in acute stroke.

You cannot, of course, cure anyone of a stroke by rolling a dice, but if these simulated results pertained to a genuine medical controversy (such as which postmenopausal women would be best advised to take hormone replacement therapy or whether breech babies should routinely be delivered by Caesarean section), how would you spot these subtle biases? The answer is you need to work through the what-ifs. What if the authors of the systematic review had changed the inclusion criteria? What if they had excluded unpublished studies? What if their 'quality weightings' had been assigned differently? What if trials of lower methodological quality had been included (or excluded)? What if all the unaccounted-for patients in a trial were assumed to have died (or been cured)?

An exploration of what-ifs is known as a *sensitivity analysis*. If you find that fiddling with the data like this in various ways makes little or no difference to the review's overall results, you can assume that the review's conclusions are relatively robust. If, however, the key findings disappear when any of the what-ifs changes, the conclusions should be expressed far more cautiously and you should hesitate before changing your practice in the light of them.

Question Five: Have the numerical results been interpreted with common sense and due regard to the broader aspects of the problem?

As the next section shows, it is easy to be phased by the figures and graphs in a systematic review. But any numerical result, however precise, accurate, 'significant', or otherwise incontrovertible, must be placed in the context of the painfully simple and (often) frustratingly general question that the review addressed. The clinician must decide how (if at all) this numerical result, *whether significant or not*, should influence the care of an individual patient.

A particularly important feature to consider when undertaking or appraising a systematic review is the external validity of included trials (see Box 9.3). A trial may be of high methodological quality and have a

---

Box 9.3 Assigning weight to trials in a systematic review

Each trial should be evaluated in terms of its:

- *methodological quality* – that is, extent to which the design and conduct are likely to have prevented systematic errors (bias) (see section 'Was systematic bias avoided or minimised?');
- *precision* – that is, a measure of the likelihood of random errors (usually depicted as the width of the confidence interval around the result);
- *external validity* – that is, the extent to which the results are generalisable or applicable to a particular target population.

(Additional aspects of 'quality' such as scientific importance, clinical importance and literary quality are rightly given great weight by peer reviewers and journal editors, but are less relevant to the systematic reviewer once the question to be addressed has been defined.)

precise and numerically impressive result, but it may, for example, have been conducted on participants under the age of 60, and hence may not apply at all to people over 75 for good physiological reasons. The inclusion in systematic reviews of irrelevant studies is guaranteed to lead to absurdities and reduce the credibility of secondary research.

Meta-analysis for the non-statistician

If I had to pick one term that exemplifies the fear and loathing felt by so many students, clinicians and consumers towards EBM, that word would be 'meta-analysis'. The meta-analysis, defined as *a statistical synthesis of the numerical results of several trials that all addressed the same question*, is the statisticians' chance to pull a double whammy on you. First, they frighten you with all the statistical tests in the individual papers, and then they use a whole new battery of tests to produce a new set of odds ratios, confidence intervals and values for significance.

As I confessed in Chapter 5, I too tend to go into panic mode at the sight of ratios, square root signs and half-forgotten Greek letters. But before you consign meta-analysis to the set of specialised techniques that you will never understand, remember two things. First, the meta-analyst may wear an anorak but he or she is *on your side*. A good meta-analysis is often easier for the non-statistician to understand than the stack of primary research papers from which it was derived, for reasons I am about to explain. Second, the underlying statistical principles used for meta-analysis are the same as the ones for any other data analysis – it's just that some of the numbers are bigger.

The first task of the meta-analyst, after following the preliminary steps for systematic review in Figure 9.1, is to decide which out of all the various outcome measures chosen by the authors of the primary studies is the best one (or ones) to use in the overall synthesis. In trials of a particular chemotherapy regimen for breast cancer, for example, some authors will have published cumulative mortality figures (i.e. the total number of people who have died to date) at cut-off points of 3 and 12 months, whereas other trials will have published 6-month, 12-month and 5-year cumulative mortality. The meta-analyst might decide to concentrate on 12-month mortality because this result can be easily extracted from all the papers. He or she may, however, decide that 3-month mortality is a clinically important end-point, and would need to write to the authors of the remaining trials asking for the raw data from which to calculate these figures.

In addition to crunching the numbers, part of the meta-analyst's job description is to tabulate relevant information on the inclusion criteria, sample size, baseline patient characteristics, withdrawal ('drop-out') rate and results of primary and secondary end-points of all the studies included. If this task has been performed properly, you will be able to compare both the methods and the results of two trials whose authors wrote up their research in different ways. Although such tables are often visually daunting, they save you having to plough through the methods sections of each paper and compare one author's tabulated results with another author's pie chart or histogram.

These days, the results of meta-analyses tend to be presented in a fairly standard form. This is partly because meta-analysts often use computer software to do the calculations for them (see the latest edition of the Cochrane Reviewers' handbook for an up-to-date menu of options [12]), and most such software packages include a standard graphics tool that presents results as illustrated in Figure 9.2. I have reproduced (with the authors' permission) this pictorial representation (colloquially known as a *forest plot* or *blobbogram*) of the pooled odds ratios of eight randomised controlled trials of therapy for depression. Each of these eight studies had compared a group receiving cognitive behaviour therapy (CBT) with a control group that received no active treatment and in whom pharmacotherapy (PHA – i.e. drug treatment) was discontinued [14]. The primary (main) outcome in this meta-analysis was relapse within 1 year.

The eight trials, each represented by the surname of the first author and the year that paper was published (e.g. 'Blackburn 1986') are listed, one below the other on the left hand side of the figure. The horizontal line corresponding to each trial shows the likelihood of relapse by 1 year in patients randomised to CBT compared to patients randomised to PHA. The 'blob' in the middle of

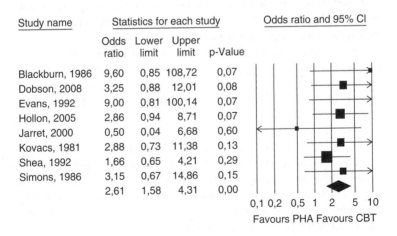

Figure 9.2 Forest plot showing long-term effects of cognitive behaviour therapy (CBT) compared with no active treatment and discontinuation of pharmacotherapy (PHA). Source: Cuijpers et al. [14]. Reproduced with permission from BMJ.

each line is the point estimate of the difference between the groups (the best single estimate of the benefit in improved relapse rate by offering CBT rather than PHA), and the width of the line represents the 95% confidence interval of this estimate (see section 'Have confidence intervals been calculated, and do the authors' conclusions reflect them?'). The key vertical line to look at, known as the *line of no effect*, is the one marking the relative risk (RR) of 1.0. Note that if the horizontal line for any trial does not cross the line of no effect, there is a 95% chance that there is a 'real' difference between the groups.

As sections 'Were preliminary statistical questions addressed?' and 'Probability and confidence' argued, if the confidence interval of the result (the horizontal line) *does* cross the line of no effect (i.e. the vertical line at RR = 1.0), that can mean *either* that there is no significant difference between the treatments, *and/or* that the sample size was too small to allow us to be confident where the true result lies. The various individual studies give point estimates of the odds ratio of CBT compared to PHA (of between 0.5 and 9.6), and the confidence intervals of some studies are so wide that they don't even fit on the graph.

Now, here comes the fun of meta-analysis. Look at the tiny diamond below all the horizontal lines. This represents the *pooled* data from all eight trials (overall RR CBT:PHA = 2.61, meaning that CBT has 2.61 times the odds of preventing relapse), with a new, much narrower, confidence interval of this RR (1.58–4.31). Because the diamond does not overlap the line of no effect, we can say that there is a statistically significant difference between the two treatments in terms of the primary end-point (relapse of depression in the first year). Now, in this example, seven of the eight trials suggested a benefit from CBT, but in none of them was the sample size large enough for that finding to be statistically significant.

Note, however, that this neat little diamond does *not* mean that you should offer CBT to every patient with depression. It has a much more limited meaning – that the *average* patient in the trials presented in this meta-analysis is likely to benefit in terms of the primary outcome (relapse of depression within a year) if they receive CBT. The choice of treatment should, of course, take into account how the patient feels about embarking on a course of CBT (see Chapter 16) and also on the relative merits of this therapy compared to *other* treatments for depression. The paper from which Figure 9.2 is taken also described a second meta-analysis that showed no significant difference between CBT and continuing antidepressant therapy, suggesting, perhaps, that patients who prefer not to have CBT may do just as well by continuing to take their tablets [14].

As this example shows, 'non-significant' trials (i.e. ones that, on their own, did not demonstrate a significant difference between treatment and control

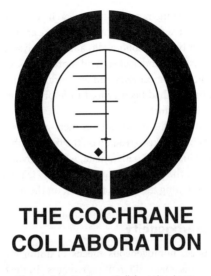

**THE COCHRANE
COLLABORATION**

Figure 9.3 Cochrane Collaboration Logo.

groups) contribute to a pooled result in a meta-analysis that *is* statistically significant. The most famous example of this, which the Cochrane Collaboration adopted as its logo (Figure 9.3), is the meta-analysis of seven trials of the effect of giving steroids to mothers who were expected to give birth prematurely [15]. Only two of the seven trials showed a statistically significant benefit (in terms of survival of the infant), but the improvement in precision (i.e. the narrowing of confidence intervals) in the pooled results, shown by the narrower width of the diamond compared with the individual lines, demonstrates the strength of the evidence in favour of this intervention. This meta-analysis showed that infants of steroid-treated mothers were 30–50% less likely to die than infants of control mothers. This example is discussed further in section 'Why are health professionals slow to adopt evidence-based practice?' in relation to changing clinicians' behaviour.

You may have worked out by now that anyone who is thinking about doing a clinical trial of an intervention should first do a meta-analysis of all the previous trials on that same intervention. In practice, researchers only occasionally do this. Dean Fergusson and colleagues of the Ottawa Health Research Institute published a cumulative meta-analysis of all randomised controlled trials carried out on the drug aprotinin in peri-operative bleeding during cardiac surgery [16]. They lined up the trials in the order they had been published, and worked out what a meta-analysis of 'all trials done so far' would have shown (had it been performed at the time). The resulting *cumulative meta-analysis* had shocking news for the research communities. The beneficial effect of aprotinin reached statistical significance after only 12 trials – that is, back in 1992. But because nobody did a meta-analysis at the time, a further 52 clinical trials were undertaken (and more may be ongoing). All these trials were scientifically unnecessary and unethical (because half the patients were denied a drug that had been proved to improve outcome). Figure 9.4 illustrates this waste of effort.

If you have followed the arguments on meta-analysis of published trial results this far, you might like to read up on the more sophisticated technique of meta-analysis of individual patient data, which provides a more accurate and precise figure for the point estimate of effect [17]. You might also like to hunt out what is becoming the classic textbook on the topic [18].

Explaining heterogeneity

In everyday language, 'homogeneous' means 'of uniform composition', and 'heterogeneous' means 'many different ingredients'. In the language of meta-analysis, homogeneity means that the results of each individual trial are compatible with the results of any of the others. Homogeneity can be estimated at a glance once the trial results have been presented in the format illustrated in Figures 9.2 and 9.5. In Figure 9.2, the lower confidence interval of every trial is below the upper confidence interval of all the others (i.e. the horizontal lines all overlap to some extent). Statistically speaking, the trials are homogeneous. Conversely, in Figure 9.4, there are some trials whose lower confidence interval is above the upper confidence interval of one or more other trials (i.e. some lines do not overlap at all). These trials may be said to be heterogeneous.

You may have spotted by now (particularly if you have already read section 'Have confidence intervals been calculated, and do the authors' conclusions reflect them?' on confidence intervals) that pronouncing a set of trials heterogeneous on the basis of whether their confidence intervals overlap is somewhat arbitrary, as the confidence interval itself is arbitrary (it can be set at 90%, 95%, 99% or indeed any other value). The definitive test involves a slightly more sophisticated statistical manoeuvre than holding a ruler up against the blobbogram. The one most commonly used is a variant of the Chi-square (χ^2) test (see Table 5.1), as the question addressed is, 'is there greater variation between the results of the trials than is compatible with the play of chance?'.

The χ^2 statistic for heterogeneity is explained in more detail by Thompson [19], who offers the following useful rule of thumb: a χ^2 statistic has, on average, a value equal to its degrees of freedom (in this case, the number of trials in the meta-analysis minus one), so a χ^2 of 7.0 for a set of 8 trials would

Ref #	Year of Publication	# Pts
6	Dec - 87	22
7	Mar-89	99
8	Apr-89	175
9	Sep-90	219
10	Oct-90	257
11	Dec-90	296
12	Jun-91	376
13	Sep-91	396
14	Dec-91	455
15	Apr-92	486
16	Jun-92	601
17	Jun-92	2385
18	Jun-92	2445
19	Nov-92	2495
20	Dec-92	2664
21	Jan-93	2754
22	Jul-93	2795
23	Aug-93	3005
24	Dec-93	3044
25	Jan-94	3146
26a	Feb-94	3201
26b	Feb-94	3342
27	Feb-94	3396
28	Apr-94	3475
29	Jul-94	3575
30	Aug-94	3668
31	Aug-94	3724
32	Oct-94	3822
33	Oct-94	3854
34	Dec-94	3882
35	Dec-94	4047
36	Feb-95	4147
37	Feb-95	4210
38	Feb-95	4240
39	Apr-95	4338
40	Jun-95	4382
41	Jun-95	4420
42	Sep-95	4450
43	Oct-95	4548
44	Oct-95	4578
45	Oct-95	4832
46	May-96	4882
47	Jul-96	4975
48	Aug-96	5023
49	Aug-96	5135
50	Oct-96	5326
51	Dec-96	5970
52	Jan-97	6008
53	Jan-97	6060
54	Aug-97	6227
55	Sep-97	6333
56	Dec-97	6376
57a	Oct-98	6442
57b	Oct-98	6507
58	Nov-98	7303
59	Aug-99	7360
60	Sep-99	7510
61	Mar-00	7593
62	Dec-00	7677
63	Dec-00	7697
64	Jan-01	7897
65	Sep-01	7952
66	Sep-01	8011
67	Jun-02	8040

Figure 9.4 Cumulative meta-analysis of randomised controlled trials of aprotinin in cardiac surgery [16]. Reproduced with permission of Clinical Trials.

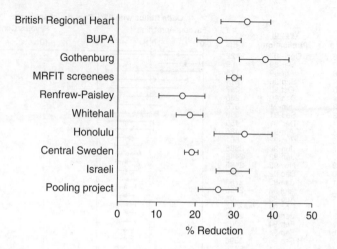

Figure 9.5 Reduction in heart disease risk by cholesterol-lowering strategies. Source: Greenhalgh [20]. Reproduced with permission of Royal College of General Practitioners.

provide no evidence of statistical heterogeneity. (In fact, it would not prove that the trials were homogeneous either, particularly because the χ^2 test has low power (see section 'Were preliminary statistical questions addressed?') to detect small but important levels of heterogeneity.)

A χ^2 value much greater than the number of trials in a meta-analysis tells us that the trials that contributed to the analysis are different in some important way from one another. There may, for example, be known differences in method (e.g. authors may have used different questionnaires to assess the symptoms of depression), or known clinical differences in the trial participants (e.g. one centre might have been a tertiary referral hospital to which all the sickest patients were referred). There may, however, be unknown or unrecorded differences between the trials which the meta-analyst can only speculate upon until he or she has extracted further details from the trials' authors. Remember: demonstrating statistical heterogeneity is a mathematical exercise and is the job of the statistician, but *explaining* this heterogeneity (i.e. looking for, and accounting for, *clinical* heterogeneity) is an interpretive exercise and requires imagination, common sense and hands-on clinical or research experience.

Figure 9.5, which is reproduced with permission from Thompson's [19] chapter on the subject, shows the results of ten trials of cholesterol-lowering strategies. The results are expressed as the percentage reduction in heart disease risk associated with each 0.6 mmol/l reduction in serum cholesterol level.

The horizontal lines represent the 95% confidence intervals of each result, and it is clear, even without being told the χ^2 statistic of 127, that the trials are highly heterogeneous.

To simply 'average out' the results of the trials in Figure 9.5 would be very misleading. The meta-analyst must return to his or her primary sources and ask, 'in what way was trial A different from trial B, and what do trials E, F and H have in common which makes their results cluster at one extreme of the figure?' In this example, a correction for the age of the trial participants reduced χ^2 from 127 to 45. In other words, most of the 'incompatibility' in the results of these trials can be explained by the fact that embarking on a strategy (such as a special diet) that successfully reduces your cholesterol level will be substantially more likely to prevent a heart attack if you are 45 than if you are 85.

This, essentially, is the essence of the grievance of Professor Hans Eysenck [21], who has constructed a vigorous and entertaining critique of the science of meta-analysis. In a world of lumpers and splitters, Eysenck is a splitter, and it offends his sense of the qualitative and the particular (see Chapter 12) to combine the results of studies that were performed on different populations in different places at different times and for different reasons.

Eysenck's reservations about meta-analysis are borne out in the infamously discredited meta-analysis that demonstrated (wrongly) that there was significant benefit to be had from giving intravenous magnesium to heart attack victims. A subsequent megatrial involving 58 000 patients (ISIS-4) failed to find any benefit whatsoever, and the meta-analysts' misleading conclusions were subsequently explained in terms of publication bias, methodological weaknesses in the smaller trials and clinical heterogeneity [22, 23]. (Incidentally, for more debate on the pros and cons of meta-analysis versus megatrials, see this recent paper [24].)

Eysenck's mathematical naiveté is embarrassing ('if a medical treatment has an effect so recondite and obscure as to require a meta-analysis to establish it, I would not be happy to have it used on me'), which is perhaps why the editors of the second edition of the 'Systematic reviews' book dropped his chapter from their collection. But I have a great deal of sympathy for the principle of his argument. As one who tends to side with the splitters, I would put Eysenck's misgivings about meta-analysis high on the list of required reading for the aspiring systematic reviewer. Indeed, I once threw my own hat into the ring when Griffin [25] published a meta-analysis of primary studies into the management of diabetes by primary health care teams. Although I have a high regard for Simon as a scientist, I felt strongly that he had not been justified in performing a mathematical summation of what I believed were very different studies all addressing slightly different questions. As I said in my commentary on his article, 'four apples and five oranges make four apples and five oranges, not nine apple and oranges' [26]. But Simon numbers himself among the lumpers, and there are plenty of people cleverer than I who have argued that he was entirely correct to analyse his data as he did. Fortunately, the two of us have agreed to differ – and on a personal level we remain friends.

New approaches to systematic review

This chapter has addressed the most commonly used approach to systematic review – synthesising trials of therapy. If you're comfortable with that, you might like to start exploring the literature on more challenging forms of systematic review – such as diagnostic studies [27] and the emerging science of systematic review of qualitative research (and mixed qualitative and quantitative studies), which I discuss in more detail in Chapter 11. For my own part, I've been working with colleagues to develop new approaches to systematic review that highlight and explore (rather than attempt to 'average out') the fundamental differences between primary studies – an approach that I think is particularly useful for developing systematic reviews in health care policy-making [28, 29]. But these relatively small-print applications are all beyond the basics, and if you're reading this book to get you through an exam, you'll probably find they aren't on the syllabus.

If you found yourself sympathising with Professor Eysenck in the previous section, you might like to look at some other theoretical critiques of systematic review. MacLure [30] has written an excellent philosophical article claiming that with its overemphasis on protocols and procedures, a conventional systematic review degrades the status of interpretive scholarly activities such as reading, writing and talking, and replaces them with a series of auditable technical tasks. This change, she claims, is partly driven by the new managerialism in research and results in 'the call-centre version of research synthesis'. I once wrote a short commentary called *Why are Cochrane Reviews so boring?*, arguing that an overly technocratic approach to data extraction and synthesis strips the *meaning* from a review [20]. But whilst this may be true and MacLure may have a point, we shouldn't throw the baby out with the bath water. Systematic review, in its place, saves lives.

References

1 Caveman A. The invited review? or, my field, from my standpoint, written by me using only my data and my ideas, and citing only my publications. Journal of Cell Science 2000;**113**(Pt 18):3125.

2 Pauling L. *How to live longer and feel better*, Portland, Oregon. Oregon State University Press. 1986;3125–3126.

3 McAlister FA, Clark HD, van Walraven C, et al. The medical review article revisited: has the science improved? Annals of Internal Medicine 1999;**131**(12):947–51.

4 Oxman AD, Guyatt GH. The science of reviewing research. Annals of the New York Academy of Sciences 1993;**703**(1):125–34.

5 Antman EM, Lau J, Kupelnick B, et al. A comparison of results of meta-analyses of randomized control trials and recommendations of clinical experts. JAMA: The Journal of the American Medical Association 1992;**268**(2):240–8.

6 Knipschild P. Systematic reviews. Some examples. BMJ: British Medical Journal 1994;**309**(6956):719–21.

7 Moher D, Liberati A, Tetzlaff J, et al. Preferred reporting items for systematic reviews and meta-analyses: the PRISMA statement. Annals of Internal Medicine 2009;**151**(4):264–9.

8 Bruins Slot KM, Berge E, Saxena R, et al. Oral anticoagulants versus antiplatelet therapy for preventing stroke and systemic embolic events in patients with atrial fibrillation. Cochrane Database of Systematic Reviews 2012, Issue 2. Art. No.: CD009538. DOI: 10.1002/14651858.CD009538.

9 Greenhalgh T, Robert G, Macfarlane F, et al. Diffusion of innovations in service organizations: systematic review and recommendations. The Milbank Quarterly 2004;**82**(4):581–629 doi: 10.1111/j.0887-378X.2004.00325.x.

10 Morrison A, Polisena J, Husereau D, et al. The effect of English-language restriction on systematic review-based meta-analyses: a systematic review of empirical studies. International Journal of Technology Assessment in Health Care 2012;**28**(2):138–44.

11 Greenhalgh T, Peacock R. Effectiveness and efficiency of search methods in systematic reviews of complex evidence: audit of primary sources. BMJ: British Medical Journal 2005;**331**(7524):1064–5.

12 Higgins JPT, Green S. *Cochrane handbook for systematic reviews of interventions version 5.1. 0 [updated March 2011]*. Oxford: The Cochrane Collaboration, 2011.

13 Counsell CE, Clarke MJ, Slattery J, et al. The miracle of DICE therapy for acute stroke: fact or fictional product of subgroup analysis? BMJ: British Medical Journal 1994;**309**(6970):1677.

14 Cuijpers P, Hollon SD, van Straten A, et al. Does cognitive behaviour therapy have an enduring effect that is superior to keeping patients on continuation pharmacotherapy? A meta-analysis. BMJ Open 2013;**3**(4) doi: 10.1136/bmjopen-2012-002542[published Online First: Epub Date].

15 Egger M, Smith GD, Altman D. *Systematic reviews in health care: meta-analysis in context*. Chichester: Wiley.com, 2008.

16 Fergusson D, Glass KC, Hutton B, et al. Randomized controlled trials of aprotinin in cardiac surgery: could clinical equipoise have stopped the bleeding? Clinical Trials 2005;**2**(3):218–32.

17 Stewart LA, Tierney JF. To IPD or not to IPD? Advantages and disadvantages of systematic reviews using individual patient data. Evaluation & the Health Professions 2002;**25**(1):76–97.

18 Borenstein M, Hedges LV, Higgins JP, et al. *Introduction to meta-analysis.* Chichester: Wiley.com, 2011.

19 Thompson SG. Why and how sources of heterogeneity should be investigated. In: Egger M, Davey Smith G, Altman DG, eds. *Systematic reviews in health care: meta-analysis in context.* London: BMJ Publications, 2001;157–175.

20 Greenhalgh T. Outside the box: why are Cochrane reviews so boring? The British Journal of General Practice 2012;**62**(600):371;157–175.

21 Eysenck H. Problems with meta-analysis. In: Chalmers I, Altman DG, eds. *Systematic reviews.* London: BMJ Publications, 1995.

22 Higgins JP, Spiegelhalter DJ. Being sceptical about meta-analyses: a Bayesian perspective on magnesium trials in myocardial infarction. International Journal of Epidemiology 2002;**31**(1):96–104.

23 Egger M, Smith GD. Misleading meta-analysis. BMJ: British Medical Journal 1995;**311**(7007):753–4.

24 Hennekens CH, DeMets D. The need for large-scale randomized evidence without undue emphasis on small trials, meta-analyses, or subgroup analyses. JAMA: The Journal of the American Medical Association 2009;**302**(21):2361–2.

25 Griffin S, Greenhalgh T. Diabetes care in general practice: meta-analysis of randomised control trials Commentary: meta-analysis is a blunt and potentially misleading instrument for analysing models of service delivery. BMJ: British Medical Journal 1998;**317**(7155):390–6.

26 Greenhalgh T. Commentary: meta-analysis is a blunt and potentially misleading instrument for analysing models of service delivery. BMJ: British Medical Journal (Clinical research ed.) 1998;**317**(7155):395–6.

27 Devillé WL, Buntinx F, Bouter LM, et al. Conducting systematic reviews of diagnostic studies: didactic guidelines. BMC Medical Research Methodology 2002;**2**(1):9.

28 Wong G, Greenhalgh T, Westhorp G, et al. RAMESES publication standards: meta-narrative reviews. BMC Med 2013;11:20 doi: 10.1186/1741-7015-11-20.

29 Wong G, Greenhalgh T, Westhorp G, et al. RAMESES publication standards: realist syntheses. BMC Med 2013;11:20 doi: 10.1186/1741-7015-11-21.

30 MacLure M. 'Clarity bordering on stupidity': where's the quality in systematic review? Journal of Education Policy 2005;**20**(4):393–416.

Chapter 10 **Papers that tell you what to do (guidelines)**

The great guidelines debate

Never was the chasm between front-line clinicians and back-room policymakers wider than in their respective attitudes to clinical guidelines. Policymakers (by which I include everyone who has a view on how medicine ought to be practised in an ideal world – including politicians, senior managers, clinical directors, academics and teachers) tend to love guidelines. Front-line clinicians (i.e. people who spend all their time seeing patients) often have a strong aversion to guidelines.

Before we carry this political hot potato any further, we need a definition of guidelines, for which the following will suffice.

> *Guidelines are systematically developed statements to assist practitioner decisions about appropriate health care for specific clinical circumstances.*

A great paper on evidence-based guidelines (what they are, how they're developed, why we need them and what the controversies are) was published recently by one of my colleagues, Dr Deborah Swinglehurst [1]. I have drawn extensively on her review when updating this chapter. One important distinction Deborah makes in her paper is between guidelines (which are usually expressed in terms of general principles and leave room for judgement within broad parameters) and protocols, which she defines as follows: 'Protocols are instructions on what to do in particular circumstances. They are similar to guidelines but include less room for individual judgement, are often produced for less experienced staff, or for use in situations where eventualities are predictable'.

How to Read a Paper: The Basics of Evidence-Based Medicine, Fifth Edition. Trisha Greenhalgh.
© 2014 John Wiley & Sons, Ltd. Published 2014 by John Wiley & Sons, Ltd.

The purposes that guidelines serve are given in Box 10.1. Clinician resistance to guidelines has a number of explanations [2–7].

- Clinical freedom ('I'm not having anyone telling me how to manage my patients'.)
- Debates amongst experts about the quality of evidence ('Well, if they can't agree among themselves … ')
- Lack of appreciation of evidence by practitioners ('That's all very well, but when I trained we were always taught to hold back on steroids for asthma'.)
- Defensive medicine ('I'll check all the tests anyway – belt and braces'.)
- Strategic and cost constraints ('We can't afford to replace the equipment'.)
- Specific practical constraints ('Where on earth did I put those guidelines'?)
- Reluctance of patients to accept procedures ('Mrs Brown insists she needs a cervical smear every year'.)
- Competing influences of other non-medical factors ('When we get the new computer system up and running … ')
- Lack of appropriate, patient-specific feedback on performance ('I seem to be treating this condition OK'.)
- Confusion ('The guideline doesn't seem to help me with the problem I'm facing'.)

The image of the medical buffoon blundering blithely through the outpatient clinic still diagnosing the same illnesses and prescribing the same drugs he (or she) learnt about at medical school 40 years previously, and never having read a paper since, knocks the 'clinical freedom' argument right out of the arena. Such hypothetical situations are grist to the mill of those who would impose 'expert guidelines' on most, if not all, medical practice and hold to account all those who fail to keep in step.

Box 10.1 Purpose of guidelines

1. To make evidence-based standards explicit and accessible (but see subsequent text: few guidelines currently in circulation are truly evidence-based).
2. To make decision making in the clinic and at the bedside easier and more objective.
3. To provide a yardstick for assessing professional performance.
4. To delineate the division of labour (e.g. between general practitioners (GPs) and consultants).
5. To educate patients and professionals about current best practice.
6. To improve the cost-effectiveness of health services.
7. To serve as a tool for external control.

But the counter argument to the excessive use, and particularly the compulsive imposition, of clinical guidelines is a powerful one, and it was expressed very eloquently some years ago by Professor J Grimley Evans [8].

> *There is a fear that in the absence of evidence clearly applicable to the case in the hand a clinician might be forced by guidelines to make use of evidence which is only doubtfully relevant, generated perhaps in a different grouping of patients in another country at some other time and using a similar but not identical treatment. This is evidence-biased medicine; it is to use evidence in the manner of the fabled drunkard who searched under the street lamp for his door key because that is where the light was, even though he had dropped the key somewhere else.*

Grimley Evans' fear, which every practising clinician shares but few can articulate, is that politicians and health service managers who have jumped on the evidence-based medicine (EBM) bandwagon will use guidelines to decree the treatment of diseases rather than of patients. They will, it is feared, make judgements about people and their illnesses subservient to published evidence that an intervention is effective 'on average'. This, and other real and perceived disadvantages of guidelines, are given in Box 10.2, which has been compiled from a number of sources [2–6]. But if you read

---

Box 10.2 Drawbacks of guidelines (real and perceived)

1. Guidelines may be intellectually suspect and reflect 'expert opinion', which may formalise unsound practice.
2. By reducing medical practice variation they may standardise to 'average' rather than best practice.
3. They might inhibit innovation and prevent individual cases from being dealt with discretely and sensitively.
4. Guidelines developed at national or regional level may not reflect local needs or have the 'ownership' of local practitioners.
5. Guidelines developed in secondary care may not reflect demographic, clinical or practical differences between this setting and the primary care setting.
6. Guidelines may produce undesirable shifts in the balance of power between different professional groups (e.g. between clinicians and academics or purchasers and providers). Hence, guideline development may be perceived as a political act.
7. Out-of-date guidelines might hold back the implementation of new research evidence.

the above-mentioned distinction between guidelines and protocols, you will probably have realised that a good guideline wouldn't *force* you to abandon common sense or judgement – it would simply flag up a recommended course of action for you to consider.

Nevertheless, even a perfect guideline can make work for the busy clinician. My friend Neal Maskrey recently sent me this quote from an article in the *Lancet*.

> We surveyed one [24-hour] acute medical take in our hospital. In a relatively quiet take, we saw 18 patients with a total of 44 diagnoses. The guidelines that the on call physician should have read, remembered and applied correctly for those conditions came to 3679 pages. This number included only NICE [UK National Institute for Health and Care Excellence], the Royal Colleges and major societies from the last 3 years. If it takes 2 min to read each page, the physician on call will have to spend 122h reading to keep abreast of the guidelines [9].

The mushrooming guidelines industry owes its success at least in part to a growing 'accountability culture' that is now (many argue) being set in statute in many countries. In the UK National Health Service, all doctors, nurses, pharmacists and other health professions now have a contractual duty to provide clinical care based on best available research evidence. Officially produced or sanctioned guidelines – such as those produced by the UK National Institute of Health and Care Excellence www.nice.org.uk – are a way of both supporting and policing that laudable goal. Whilst the medicolegal implications of 'official' guidelines have rarely been tested in the UK, courts in North America have ruled that guideline developers can be held liable for faulty guidelines. More worryingly, a US court recently refused to accept adherence to an evidence-based guideline (which advised doctors to share the inherent uncertainty associated with prostate-specific antigen (PSA) testing in asymptomatic middle-aged men, and make a shared decision on whether the test was worth doing) as defence by a doctor being sued for missing an early prostate cancer in an unlucky 53-year-old [10].

How can we help ensure that evidence-based guidelines are followed?

Two of the leading international authorities on the thorny topic of implementation of clinical guidelines are Richard Grol and Jeremy Grimshaw. In one early study by Grol's team, the main factors associated with successfully following a guideline or protocol were the practitioners' perception that it was uncontroversial (68% compliance vs 35% if it was perceived to be controversial), evidence-based (71% vs 57% if not), contained explicit recommendations (67% vs 36% if the recommendations were vague) and required no change to existing routines (67% vs 44% if a major change was recommended) [7].

Another early paper, by Grimshaw and Russell [11], summarised in Table 10.1, showed that the probability of a guideline being effectively followed depended on three factors:

(a) the development strategy (where and how the guideline was produced);
(b) the dissemination strategy (how it was brought to the attention of clinicians); and
(c) the implementation strategy (how the clinician was prompted and supported to follow the guideline, including organisational issues).

In terms of the development strategy, as Table 10.1 shows, the most effective guidelines are developed locally by the people who are going to use them, introduced as part of a specific educational intervention, and implemented via a patient-specific prompt that appears at the time of the consultation. The importance of ownership (i.e. the feeling by those being asked to play by new rules that they have been involved in drawing up those rules) is surely self-evident. There is also an extensive management theory literature to support the common-sense notion that professionals will oppose changes that they perceive as threatening to their livelihood (i.e. income), self-esteem, sense of competence or autonomy. It stands to reason, therefore, that involving health professionals in setting the standards against which they are going to be judged generally produces greater changes in patient outcomes than occur if they are not involved.

Table 10.1 Classification of clinical guidelines in terms of probability of being effective

Probability of being effective	Development strategy	Dissemination strategy	Implementation strategy
High	Internal	Specific educational intervention (e.g. problem-based learning package)	Patient-specific reminder at time of consultation
Above average	Intermediate	Continuing education (e.g. lecture)	Patient-specific feedback
Below average	External, local	Mailing targeted groups	General feedback
Low	External, national	Publication in journal	General reminder

Source: Grimshaw and Russell [11]. Reproduced with permission of Elsevier.

Grimshaw's conclusions from this early paper were initially misinterpreted by some people as implying that there was no place for nationally developed guidelines, because only locally developed ones had any impact. In fact, whilst local adoption and ownership is undoubtedly crucial to the success of a guideline programme, local teams produce more robust guidelines if they draw on the range of national and international resources of evidence-based recommendations and use this as their starting point [12].

Input from local teams is not about reinventing the wheel in terms of summarising the evidence, but to take account of local practicalities when operationalising the guideline [12]. For example, a nationally produced guideline about epilepsy care might recommend an epilepsy specialist nurse in every district. But in one district, the health care teams might have advertised for such a nurse but failed to recruit one. So the 'local input' might be about how best to provide what the epilepsy nurse would have provided, in the absence of a person in the post.

In terms of dissemination and implementation of guidelines, Grimshaw's team [13] published a comprehensive systematic review of strategies intended to improve doctors' implementation of guidelines in 2005.

The findings confirmed the general principle that clinicians are not easily influenced, but that efforts to increase guideline use are often effective to some extent. Specifically:

- improvements were shown in the intended direction of the intervention in 86% of comparisons – but the effect was generally small in magnitude;
- simple reminders were the intervention most consistently observed to be effective;
- educational outreach programmes (e.g. visiting doctors in their clinics) only led to modest effects on implementation success – and were very expensive compared to less intensive approaches;
- dissemination of educational materials led to modest but potentially important effects (and of similar magnitude to more intensive interventions);
- multifaceted interventions were not necessarily more effective than single interventions;
- nothing could be concluded from most primary studies about the cost-effectiveness of the intervention.

Grimshaw et al.'s 2005 review reversed some previous 'received wisdom', which was probably the result of publication bias in trials of implementation strategies. Contrary to what I said in the first and second editions of this book, for example, expensive complex interventions aimed at improving the implementation of guidelines by doctors are generally no more effective than simple, cheaper, well-targeted ones. Only 27% of the intervention studies reviewed by Grimshaw's team were considered to be based (either implicitly or explicitly) on an explicit theory of change – in other words, the researchers in such studies generally did not base the design of their intervention on a properly articulated mechanism of action ('A is intended to lead to B which is intended to lead to C').

In a separate paper, Grimshaw's team [14] argued strongly that research into implementing guidelines should become more theory-driven. That recommendation inspired a significant stream of research, which has been summarised in a review article by Eccles and team [15] and in a systematic review of theory-driven guideline development strategies by Davies and colleagues [14]. In short, applying behaviour change theories appears to improve uptake of guidelines by clinicians – but is not a guarantee of success, for all the reasons I discuss in Chapter 15 [16].

One of Grimshaw's most important contributions to EBM was to set up a special subgroup of the Cochrane Collaboration to review and summarise emerging research on the use of guidelines and other related issues in improving professional practice. You can find details of the Effective Practice and Organisation of Care (EPOC) Group on the Cochrane website (http://www .epoc.cochrane.org/). The EPOC database now lists thousands of primary studies and over 75 systematic reviews on the general theme of getting research evidence into practice.

Ten questions to ask about a clinical guideline

Swinglehurst [1] rightly points out that all the song and dance about encouraging clinicians to follow guidelines is only justified if the guideline is worth following in the first place. Sadly, not all of them are. She suggests two aspects of a good guideline – the content (e.g. whether it is based on a comprehensive and rigorous systematic review of the evidence) and the process (how the guideline was put together). I would add a third aspect – the presentation of the guideline (how appealing it is to the busy clinician and how easy it is to follow).

Like all published articles, guidelines would be easier to evaluate on all these counts if they were presented in a standardised format, and an international standard (the Appraisal of Guidelines for Research and Evaluation (AGREE) instrument) for developing, reporting and presenting guidelines was recently published [17]. Box 10.3 offers a pragmatic checklist, based partly on the work of the AGREE group, for structuring your assessment of a clinical guideline; and Box 10.4 reproduces the revised AGREE criteria in full. Because few published guidelines currently follow such a format, you will probably have to scan the full text for answers to the questions given here. In preparing this list

Box 10.3 Outline framework for assessing a clinical guideline (see also Appendix 1)

- *Objective*: the primary objective of the guideline, including the health problem and the targeted patients, providers and settings
- *Options*: the clinical practice options considered in formulating the guideline
- *Outcomes*: significant health and economic outcomes considered in comparing alternative practices
- *Evidence*: how and when evidence was gathered, selected and synthesised
- *Values*: disclosure of how values were assigned to potential outcomes of practice options and who participated in the process
- *Benefits, harms and costs*: the type and magnitude of benefits, harms and costs expected for patients from guideline implementation
- *Recommendations*: summary of key recommendations
- *Validation*: report of any external review, comparison with other guidelines or clinical testing of guideline use
- *Sponsors and stakeholders*: disclosure of the persons who developed, funded or endorsed the guideline

Box 10.4 The six domains of the AGREE II instrument (see reference [16])

Domain 1: Scope and purpose
1. The overall objective(s) of the guideline is(are) specifically described.
2. The health question(s) covered by the guideline is(are) specifically described.
3. The population to whom the guideline is meant to apply are specifically described.

Domain 2: Stakeholder involvement
1. The guideline development group includes individuals from all the relevant professional groups.
2. The views and preferences of the target population have been sought.
3. The target users of the guideline are clearly defined.

Domain 3: Rigour of development
1. Systematic methods were used to search for evidence.
2. The criteria for selecting the evidence are clearly described.
3. The strengths and limitations of the body of evidence are clearly described.
4. The methods used for formulating the recommendations are clearly described.

5. The health benefits, side effects and risks have been considered in formulating the recommendations.
6. There is an explicit link between the recommendations and the supporting evidence.
7. The guideline has been externally reviewed by experts prior to its publication.
8. A procedure for updating the guideline is provided.

Domain 4: Clarity and presentation
1. The recommendations are specific and unambiguous.
2. The different options for management of the condition or health issue are clearly presented.
3. Key recommendations are easily identifiable.

Domain 5: Applicability
1. The guideline provides advice or tools to support its implementation.
2. The guideline describes facilitators of, and barriers to, adoption.
3. Potential resource implications of applying the recommendations have been considered.
4. The guideline presents monitoring or auditing criteria.

Domain 6: Editorial independence
1. The views of the funding body have not influenced the content of the guideline.
2. Competing interests of members of the guideline development group have been recorded and addressed.

I have drawn on many of the other articles referenced in this chapter as well as the relatively new AGREE instrument.

Question One: Did the preparation and publication of this guideline involve a significant conflict of interest?

I will resist labouring the point, but a drug company that makes hormone replacement therapy or a research professor whose life's work has been spent perfecting this treatment might be tempted to recommend it for wider indications than the average clinician. Much has been written about the 'medicalisation' of human experience (are energetic children with a short attention span 'hyperactive'; should women with low sex drive be offered 'treatment', etc.). A guideline may be evidence-based, but the problem it addresses will have been constructed by a team that views the world in a particular way.

Question Two: Is the guideline concerned with an appropriate topic, and does it state clearly the target group it applies to?

Key questions in relation to choice of topic, reproduced from an article published a few years ago in the *British Medical Journal* [18], are given in Box 10.5.

The Grimley Evans quote on page 137 begs the question 'To whom does this guideline apply?'. If the evidence related to people aged 18–65 with no comorbidity (i.e. with nothing else wrong with them except the disease being considered), it might not apply to your patient. Sometimes this means you will need to reject it outright, but more commonly, you will have to exercise your judgement in assessing its transferability.

Question Three: Did the guideline development panel include [a] an expert in the topic area; [b] a specialist in the methods of secondary research (e.g. meta-analyst, health economist) and [c] a person affected by the condition?

If a clinical guideline has been prepared entirely by a panel of internal 'experts', you should, paradoxically, look at it particularly critically as researchers have been shown to be less objective in appraising evidence in their own field of expertise than in someone else's. The involvement of an outsider (an expert in guideline development rather than in the particular clinical topic) to act as arbiter and methodological adviser should make the process more objective. But as Gabbay and his team [19] showed in an elegant qualitative study, the hard-to-measure expertise (what might be called *embodied knowledge*) of front-line clinicians (in this case, GPs) contributed crucially to the development of workable local guidelines. But all the objective expertise in the world is no substitute for having

---

Box 10.5 Key questions on choice of topic for guideline development (see reference [17])

- Is the topic high volume, high risk, and high cost?
- Are there large or unexplained variations in practice?
- Is the topic important in terms of the process and outcome of patient care?
- Is there potential for improvement?
- Is the investment of time and money likely to be repaid?
- Is the topic likely to hold the interest of team members?
- Is consensus likely?
- Will change benefit patients?
- Can change be implemented?

the condition in question yourself, and emerging evidence suggests that patients and carers bring a crucial third perspective to the guideline development process [20].

Question Four: Have the subjective judgements of the development panel been made explicit, and are they justified?

Guideline development is not just a technical process of finding evidence, appraising it and turning it into recommendations. Recommendations also require judgements (relating to personal or social values, ethical principles, etc.). As the UK National Institute for Health and Care Excellence (NICE) has stated (see www.nice.org.uk), it is right and proper for guideline developers to take account of the 'ethical principles, preferences, culture and aspirations that should underpin the nature and extent of care provided by the National Health Service'. Swinglehurst [1] suggests four sub-questions to ask about these subjective judgements.

- What *guiding principles* have been used to decide how effective an intervention must be (compared with its potential harms) before its recommendation is considered?
- What *values* have underpinned the panel's decisions about which guideline developments to prioritise?
- What is the *ethical framework* to which guideline developers are working – in particular relating to matters of distributive justice ('rationing')?
- Where there was disagreement between guideline developers, what *explicit processes* have been used to resolve such disagreements?

Question Five: Have all the relevant data been scrutinised and rigorously evaluated?

The academic validity of guidelines depends (among other things) on whether they are supported by high-quality primary research studies, and on how strong the evidence from those studies is. At the most basic level, was the literature analysed at all, or are these guidelines simply a statement of the preferred practice of a selected panel of experts (i.e. consensus guidelines)? If the literature was looked at, was a systematic search performed, and if so, did it broadly follow the method described in section 'Evaluating systematic reviews'? Were all papers unearthed by the search included, or was an explicit scoring system (such as GRADE [21]) used to reject those of poor methodological quality and give those of high quality the extra weight they deserved?

Up-to-date systematic reviews should ideally be the raw material for guideline development. But in many cases, a search for rigorous and relevant research on which to base guidelines proves fruitless, and the authors, unavoidably, resort to 'best available' evidence or expert opinion.

Question Six: Has the evidence been properly synthesised, and are the guideline's conclusions in keeping with the data on which they are based?
Another key determinant of the validity of a guideline is how the different studies contributing to it have been pulled together (that is, synthesised) in the context of the clinical and policy needs being addressed. For one thing, a systematic review and meta-analysis might have been appropriate, and if the latter, issues of probability and confidence should have been dealt with acceptably (see section 'Summing up').

But systematic reviews don't exist (and never will exist) to cover every eventuality in clinical decision-making and policymaking. In many areas, especially complex ones, the opinion of experts is still the best 'evidence' around, and in such cases guideline developers should adopt rigorous methods to ensure that it isn't just the voice of the expert who talks for longest in the meetings that drives the recommendations. Formal guideline development groups usually have an explicit set of methods – see, for example, this paper from the UK NICE [22].

A recent analysis of three 'evidence-based' guidelines for obstructive sleep apnoea found that they made very different recommendations despite being based on an almost identical set of primary studies. The main reason for the discrepancy was that experts tended to rank studies from their own country more highly [23]!

Question Seven: Does the guideline address variations in medical practice and other controversial areas (e.g. optimum care in response to genuine or perceived underfunding)?
It would be foolish to make dogmatic statements about ideal practice without reference to what actually goes on in the real world. There are many instances where some practitioners are marching to an altogether different tune from the rest of us (see section 'Why do people sometimes groan when you mention evidence-based medicine?'), and a good guideline should face such realities head on rather than hoping that the misguided minority will fall into step by default.

Another thorny issue that guidelines should tackle head-on is where essential compromises should be made if financial constraints preclude 'ideal' practice. If the ideal, for example, is to offer all patients with significant coronary artery disease a bypass operation (at the time of writing it isn't, but never mind), and the health service can only afford to fund 20% of such procedures, who should be pushed to the front of the queue?

Question Eight: Is the guideline clinically relevant, comprehensive and flexible?
In other words, is it written from the perspective of the practising doctor, nurse, midwife, physiotherapist, and so on, and does it take account of the type of patients he or she is likely to see, and in what circumstances?

Perhaps the most frequent source of trouble here is when guidelines developed in secondary care and intended for use in hospital outpatients (who tend to be at the sicker end of the clinical spectrum) are passed on to the primary health care team with the intention of their being used in the primary care setting, where, in general, patients are less ill and may well need fewer investigations and less aggressive management. This issue is discussed in section 'Validating diagnostic tests against a gold standard' in relation to the different utilities of diagnostic and screening tests in different populations.

Guidelines should cover all, or most, clinical eventualities. What if the patient is intolerant of the recommended medication? What if you can't send off all the recommended blood tests? What if the patient is very young, very old, or suffers from a coexisting illness? These, after all, are the patients who prompt most of us to reach for our guidelines; while the more 'typical' patient tends to be managed without recourse to written instructions. Recent work by Shekelle's team [2] has added a crucial factor – multimorbidity – to the barriers to following guidelines: sometimes the patient has a condition that makes the standard recommended therapy impossible to apply. It follows that guideline developers should routinely consider common comorbidities when they set their recommendations.

Flexibility is a particularly important consideration for national and regional bodies who set themselves up to develop guidelines. As noted earlier, ownership of guidelines by the people who are intended to use them locally is crucial to whether the guidelines are actually used. If there is no free rein for practitioners to adapt them to meet local needs and priorities, a set of guidelines will probably never get taken out of the drawer.

Question Nine: Does the guideline take into account what is acceptable to, affordable by and practically possible for patients?

There is an apocryphal story of a physician in the 1940s (a time when no effective medicines for high blood pressure were available), who discovered that restricting the diet of hypertensive patients to plain, boiled, unsalted rice dramatically reduced their blood pressure and also reduced the risk of stroke. The story goes, however, that the diet made the patients so miserable that many of them committed suicide.

This is an extreme example, but within the past few years I have seen guidelines for treating constipation in the elderly that offered no alternative to the combined insults of large amounts of bran and twice-daily suppositories. Small wonder that the district nurses who were issued with them (for whom I have a good deal of respect) have gone back to giving castor oil.

For a further discussion on how to incorporate the needs and priorities of patients in guideline development, see a recent review [20].

148   **How to read a paper**

Question Ten: Does the guideline include recommendations for its own dissemination, implementation and regular review?
Given the well-documented gap between what is known to be good practice and what actually happens (see preceding text), and the barriers to the successful implementation of guidelines discussed in section 'How can we help ensure that evidence-based guidelines are followed?', it would be in the interests of those who develop guidelines to suggest methods of maximising their use. If this objective were included as standard in the 'Guidelines for good guidelines', the guideline writers' output would probably include fewer ivory tower recommendations and more that are plausible, possible and capable of being explained to patients. Having said that, one very positive development in EBM since I wrote the first edition of this book is the change in guideline developers' attitudes: they now often take responsibility for linking their outputs to clinicians (and patients) in the real world and for reviewing and updating their recommendations periodically.

References

1 Swinglehurst D. Evidence-based guidelines: the theory and the practice. Evidence-Based Healthcare and Public Health 2005;9(4):308–14.
2 Shekelle P, Woolf S, Grimshaw JM, et al. Developing clinical practice guidelines: reviewing, reporting, and publishing guidelines; updating guidelines; and the emerging issues of enhancing guideline implementability and accounting for comorbid conditions in guideline development. Implementation Science 2012; 7(1):62.
3 Gurses AP, Marsteller JA, Ozok AA, et al. Using an interdisciplinary approach to identify factors that affect clinicians' compliance with evidence-based guidelines. Critical Care Medicine 2010;38:S282–91.
4 Gagliardi AR, Brouwers MC, Palda VA, et al. How can we improve guideline use? A conceptual framework of implementability. Implementation Science 2011;6(1):26.
5 Evans-Lacko S, Jarrett M, McCrone P, et al. Facilitators and barriers to implementing clinical care pathways. BMC Health Services Research 2010;10(1):182.
6 Michie S, Johnston M. Changing clinical behaviour by making guidelines specific. BMJ: British Medical Journal 2004;328(7435):343.
7 Grol R, Dalhuijsen J, Thomas S, et al. Attributes of clinical guidelines that influence use of guidelines in general practice: observational study. BMJ: British Medical Journal 1998;317(7162):858–61.
8 Evans JG. Evidence-based and evidence-biased medicine. Age and Ageing 1995; 24(6):461–3.
9 Allen D, Harkins K. Too much guidance? The Lancet 2005;365(9473):1768.
10 Merenstein D. Winners and losers. JAMA: The Journal of the American Medical Association 2004;291(1):15–6.

11 Grimshaw JM, Russell IT. Effect of clinical guidelines on medical practice: a systematic review of rigorous evaluations. The Lancet 1993;342(8883):1317–22.

12 Harrison MB, Légaré F, Graham ID, et al. Adapting clinical practice guidelines to local context and assessing barriers to their use. Canadian Medical Association Journal 2010;182(2):E78–84.

13 Grimshaw J, Thomas R, MacLennan G, et al. Effectiveness and efficiency of guideline dissemination and implementation strategies. International Journal of Technology Assessment in Health Care 2005;21(01):149.

14 Eccles M, Grimshaw J, Walker A, et al. Changing the behavior of healthcare professionals: the use of theory in promoting the uptake of research findings. Journal of Clinical Epidemiology 2005;58(2):107–12.

15 Eccles MP, Grimshaw JM, MacLennan G, et al. Explaining clinical behaviors using multiple theoretical models. Implementation Science 2012;7:99.

16 Davies P, Walker AE, Grimshaw JM. A systematic review of the use of theory in the design of guideline dissemination and implementation strategies and interpretation of the results of rigorous evaluations. Implementation Science 2010;5:14.

17 Brouwers MC, Kho ME, Browman GP, et al. AGREE II: advancing guideline development, reporting and evaluation in health care. Canadian Medical Association Journal 2010;182(18):E839–42.

18 Thomson R, Lavender M, Madhok R. How to ensure that guidelines are effective. BMJ: British Medical Journal 1995;311(6999):237–42.

19 Gabbay J, May Al. Evidence based guidelines or collectively constructed "mindlines?" Ethnographic study of knowledge management in primary care. BMJ: British Medical Journal 2004;329(7473):1013.

20 Boivin A, Currie K, Fervers B, et al. Patient and public involvement in clinical guidelines: international experiences and future perspectives. Quality and Safety in Health Care 2010;19(5):1–4.

21 Guyatt G, Oxman AD, Akl EA, et al. GRADE guidelines: 1. Introduction – GRADE evidence profiles and summary of findings tables. Journal of Clinical Epidemiology 2011;64(4):383–94.

22 Hill J, Bullock I, Alderson P. A summary of the methods that the National Clinical Guideline Centre uses to produce clinical guidelines for the National Institute for Health and Clinical Excellence. Annals of Internal Medicine 2011;154(11):752–7.

23 Aarts MC, van der Heijden GJ, Rovers MM, et al. Remarkable differences between three evidence-based guidelines on management of obstructive sleep apnea-hypopnea syndrome. The Laryngoscope 2013;123(1):283–91.

Chapter 11 Papers that tell you what things cost (economic analyses)

What is economic analysis?

An economic analysis can be defined as *one that involves the use of analytical techniques to define choices in resource allocation.* Most of what I have to say on this subject comes from advice prepared by Professor Michael Drummond's team [1] for authors and reviewers of economic analyses as well as the excellent pocket-sized summary by Jefferson et al. [2], both of which emphasise the importance of setting the economic questions about a paper in the context of the overall quality and relevance of the study (see section 'Ten questions to ask about an economic analysis').

The first economic evaluation I ever remember was a TV advertisement in which the pop singer Cliff Richard tried to persuade a housewife that the most expensive brand of washing-up liquid on the market 'actually works out cheaper'. It was, apparently, stronger on stains, softer on the hands and produced more bubbles per penny than 'a typical cheap liquid'. Although I was only nine at the time, I was unconvinced. Which 'typical cheap liquid' was the product being compared with? How much stronger on stains was it? Why should the effectiveness of a washing-up liquid be measured in terms of bubbles produced rather than plates cleaned?

Forgive me for sticking with this trivial example, but I'd like to use it to illustrate the four main types of economic evaluation that you will find in the literature (see Table 11.1 for the conventional definitions).

- *Cost-minimisation analysis*: '"Sudso" costs 47 p per bottle whereas "Jiffo" costs 63 p per bottle'.
- *Cost-effectiveness analysis*: '"Sudso" gives you 15 extra clean plates per wash than "Jiffo"'.
- *Cost–utility analysis*: 'In terms of quality-adjusted homemaker hours (a composite score reflecting time and effort needed to scrub plates clean, and

How to Read a Paper: The Basics of Evidence-Based Medicine, Fifth Edition. Trisha Greenhalgh.
© 2014 John Wiley & Sons, Ltd. Published 2014 by John Wiley & Sons, Ltd.

hand roughness caused by the liquid), "Sudso" provides 29 units per pound spent, whereas "Jiffo" provides 23 units'.

- *Cost–benefit analysis*: 'The net overall cost (reflecting direct cost of the product, indirect cost of time spent washing up, and estimated financial value of a clean plate relative to a slightly grubby one) of "Sudso" per day is 7.17p, while that of "Jiffo" is 9.32p'.

You should be able to see immediately that the most sensible analysis to use in this example is cost-effectiveness analysis. Cost-minimisation analysis (see Table 11.1) is inappropriate as 'Sudso' and 'Jiffo' do not have identical effectiveness. Cost–utility analysis is unnecessary because, in this example, we are interested in very little else apart from the number of plates cleaned per unit of washing-up liquid – in other words, our outcome has only one important dimension. Cost–benefit analysis is, in this example, an absurdly complicated way of telling you that 'Sudso' cleans more plates per penny.

There are, however, many situations where health professionals, particularly those who purchase health care from real cash-limited budgets, must choose between interventions for a host of different conditions whose outcomes (such as cases of measles prevented, increased mobility after a hip replacement, reduced risk of death from heart attack or likelihood of giving birth to a live baby) cannot be directly compared with one another. Controversy surrounds not just how these comparisons should be made (see section 'How can we help ensure that evidence-based guidelines are followed?'), but also who should make them, and to whom the decision-makers for the 'rationing' of health care should be accountable. These essential, fascinating and frustrating questions are beyond the scope of this book, but if you are interested I recommend a recent book by Donaldson and Mitton [3].

Measuring costs and benefits of health interventions

A few years ago, I was taken to hospital to have my appendix removed. From the hospital's point of view, the cost of my care included my board and lodging for 5 days, a proportion of doctors' and nurses' time, drugs and dressings and investigations (blood tests and a scan). Other *direct costs* (see Box 11.1) included my general practitioner's time for attending to me in the middle of the night and the cost of the petrol my husband used when visiting me (not to mention the grapes and flowers).

In addition to this, there were the *indirect* costs of my loss in productivity. I was off work for 3 weeks, and my domestic duties were temporarily divided between various friends, neighbours and a nice young girl from a nanny agency. And, from my point of view, there were several *intangible* costs, such as discomfort, loss of independence, the allergic rash I developed on

Table 11.1 Types of economic analysis

Type of analysis	Outcome measure	Conditions of use	Example
Cost-minimisation analysis	No outcome measure	Used when the effect of both interventions is known (or may be assumed) to be identical	Comparing the price of a brand name drug with that of its generic equivalent if bioequivalence has been demonstrated
Cost-effectiveness analysis	Natural units (e.g. life-years gained)	Used when the effect of the interventions can be expressed in terms of one main variable	Comparing two preventive treatments for an otherwise fatal condition
Cost-utility analysis	Utility units (e.g. quality adjusted life years)	Used when the effect of the interventions on health status has two or more important dimensions (e.g. benefits and side effects of drugs)	Comparing the benefits of two treatments for varicose veins in terms of surgical result, cosmetic appearance and risk of serious adverse event (e.g. pulmonary embolus)
Cost–benefit analysis	Monetary units (e.g. estimated cost of loss in productivity)	Used when it is desirable to compare an intervention for this condition with an intervention for a different condition	For a purchasing authority, to decide whether to fund a heart transplantation programme or a stroke rehabilitation ward

Box 11.1 Examples of costs and benefits of health interventions

Costs	Benefits
Direct	**Economic**
'Board and lodging'	Prevention of expensive-to-treat illness
Drugs, dressings, etc	Avoidance of hospital admission
Investigations	Return to paid work
Staff salaries	
	Clinical
Indirect	Postponement of death or disability
Work days lost	Relief of pain, nausea, breathlessness, etc
Value of "unpaid" work	Improved vision, hearing, muscular strength, etc
Intangible	**Quality of life**
Pain and suffering	Increased mobility and independence
Social stigma	Improved wellbeing
	Release from sick role

the medication and the cosmetically unsightly scar that I now carry on my abdomen.

As Box 11.1 shows, these direct, indirect and intangible costs constitute one side of the cost–benefit equation. On the benefit side, the operation greatly increased my chances of staying alive. In addition, I had a nice rest from work, and, to be honest, I rather enjoyed all the attention and sympathy. (Note that the 'social stigma' of appendicitis can be a positive one. I would be less likely to brag about my experience if my hospital admission had been precipitated by, say, an epileptic fit or a nervous breakdown, which have negative social stigmata).

In the appendicitis example, few patients would perceive much freedom of choice in deciding to opt for the operation. But most health interventions do not concern definitive procedures for acutely life-threatening diseases. Most of us can count on developing at least one chronic, disabling and progressive condition such as ischaemic heart disease, high blood pressure, arthritis, chronic bronchitis, cancer, rheumatism, prostatic hypertrophy or diabetes. At some stage, almost all of us will be forced to decide whether having a routine operation, taking a particular drug or making a compromise in our lifestyle (reducing our alcohol intake or sticking to a cholesterol-lowering diet) is 'worth it'.

It is fine for informed individuals to make choices about their own care by gut reaction ('I'd rather live with my hernia than be cut open', or 'I know about the risk of thrombosis but I want to continue to smoke and stay on the [contraceptive] Pill'). But when the choices are about other people's care, personal values and prejudices are the last thing that should enter the equation. Most of us would want the planners and policymakers to use objective, explicit and defensible criteria when making decisions such as, 'No, Mrs Brown may not have a kidney transplant'.

One important way of addressing the 'what's it worth?' question for a given health state (such as having poorly controlled diabetes or asthma) is to ask someone in that state how they feel. A number of questionnaires that attempt to measure overall health status, such as the Nottingham Health Profile, the SF-36 general health questionnaire (widely used in the UK) and the McMaster Health Utilities Index Questionnaire (popular in north America), have been developed. For an overview of all these, see this reference textbook [4].

In some circumstances, disease-specific measures of well-being are more valid than general measures. For example, answering 'yes' to the question, 'do you get very concerned about the food you are eating?' might indicate anxiety in someone without diabetes but normal self-care attitudes in someone with diabetes [5]. There has also been an upsurge of interest in *patient-specific* measures of quality of life, to allow different patients to place different values on particular aspects of their health and well-being. When quality of life is being analysed form the point of view of the patient, this is a sensible and humane approach. However, the health economist tends to make decisions about groups of patients or populations, in which case patient-specific, and even disease-specific, measures of quality of life have limited relevance. If you would like to get up to speed in the ongoing debate on how to measure health-related quality of life, take time to look up some of the references listed at the end of this chapter [4, 6–8].

The authors of standard instruments (such as the SF-36) for measuring quality of life have often spent years ensuring they are valid (i.e. they measure what we think they are measuring), reliable (they do so every time), and responsive to change (i.e. if an intervention improves or worsens the patient's health, the scale will reflect that). For this reason, you should be highly suspicious of a paper that eschews these standard instruments in favour of the authors' own rough-and-ready scale ('functional ability was classified as good, moderate or poor according to the clinician's overall impression', or, 'we asked patients to score both their pain and their overall energy level from one to ten, and added the results together'). Note also that even instruments that have apparently been well validated often do not stand up to rigorous evaluation of their psychometric validity [8].

Another way of addressing the 'what's it worth?' of particular health states is through *health state preference values* – that is, the value which, in a hypothetical situation, a healthy person would place on a particular deterioration in their health, or which a sick person would place on a return to health [9]. There are three main methods of assigning such values.

- *Rating scale measurements*: the respondent is asked to make a mark on a fixed line, labelled, for example, 'perfect health' at one end and 'death' at the other, to indicate where he or she would place the state in question (e.g. being wheelchair-bound from arthritis of the hip).

- *Time trade-off measurements*: the respondent is asked to consider a particular health state (e.g. infertility) and estimate how many of their remaining years in full health they would sacrifice to be 'cured' of the condition.

- *Standard gamble measurements*: the respondent is asked to consider the choice between living for the rest of their life in a particular health state and taking a 'gamble' (e.g. an operation) with a given odds of success, which would return them to full health if it succeeded but kill them if it failed. The odds are then varied to see at what point the respondent decides the gamble is not worth taking.

The quality-adjusted life-year or QALY can be calculated by multiplying the preference value for that state with the time the patient is likely to spend in that state. The results of cost–benefit analyses are usually expressed in terms of 'cost per QALY', some examples of which are shown in Box 11.2 [10–15]. The absolute cost per QALY is sometimes less important in decision-making than how much the cost per QALY differs between an old, inexpensive therapy and a new, expensive one. The new drug may be only marginally more effective but many times the price! The value used to compare whether the benefit is 'worth it' is known as the incremental cost-effectiveness ratio or ICER. A good example of this is the recent introduction of dabigatran (an expensive anticoagulant but one that is less hassle for the patient than warfarin, as it involves fewer blood tests), whose ICER compared to warfarin has been estimated at £13 957 [16].

Until a few years ago, one of my many 'committee jobs' was sitting on the Appraisals Committee of NICE – the UK National Institute for Health and Care Excellence, which advises the Department of Health on the cost-effectiveness of medicines. It is very rare for the members of that multi-disciplinary committee to get through a discussion on whether to recommend funding a controversial drug without major differences of opinion surfacing and emotions rising – and, in general, high-quality QALY data tend to generate light rather than heat in such discussions. On the one hand, any measure of health state preference values is a reflection of the preferences and prejudices of the individuals who contributed to its

---

Box 11.2 Cost per QALY (see references [10–15])

Note that these are 2013 prices, so the absolute values are no longer valid; they nevertheless provide useful <u>relative</u> values for example conditions.

Statin therapy in chronic kidney disease (where baseline cardiovascular risk is high)	£1073
Statin therapy in chronic kidney disease (where baseline cardiovascular risk is low)	£98 000
Early transfer to specialist neuroscience centre for acute brain injury	£11 000
Support for lifestyle change in type 2 diabetes	£6736
Treatment of hepatitis C virus in injecting drug users	£6803
Breast reduction surgery in women with large, heavy breasts	£1054
Nicotine replacement therapies for smoking cessation	£973–£2918
Counselling for smoking cessation	£440–£1319
Telehealth in older people with multi-morbidity	£88 000

---

development. Indeed, it is possible to come up with different values for QALYs depending on how the questions from which health state preference values are derived were posed [17].

As medical ethicist John Harris has pointed out, QALYs are, like the society which produces them, inherently ageist, sexist, racist and loaded against those with permanent disabilities (because even a complete cure of an unrelated condition would not restore the individual to 'perfect health'). Furthermore, QALYs distort our ethical instincts by focusing our minds on life-years rather than people's lives. A disabled premature infant in need of an intensive care cot will, argues Harris, be allocated more resources than it deserves in comparison with a 50-year-old woman with cancer because the infant, were it to survive, would have so many more life years to quality-adjust [18].

There is an increasingly confusing array of alternatives to the QALY [4, 6, 19, 20]. Some of the ones that were in vogue when this book went to press include:

- Healthy Years Equivalent or HYE, a QALY-type measure that incorporates the individual's likely improvement or deterioration in health status in the future;

- Willingness to Pay (WTP) or Willingness to Accept (WTA), measures of how much people would be prepared to pay to gain certain benefits or avoid certain problems;
- Disability-Adjusted Life Year or DALY, used mainly in the developing world to assess the overall burden of chronic disease and deprivation – an increasingly used measure that is not without its critics; and, perhaps most bizarrely
- TWiST (time spent without symptoms of disease and toxicity of treatment) and Q-TWiST (quality-adjusted TWiST)!

My personal advice on all these measures is to look carefully at what goes into the number that is supposed to be an 'objective' indicator of a person's (or population's) health status, and at how the different measures might differ according to different disease states. In my view, they all have potential uses but none of them is an absolute or incontrovertible measure of health or illness! (Note, also, that I do not claim to be an expert on any of these measures or on how to calculate them – which is why I have offered a generous list of additional references at the end of this chapter).

There is, however, another form of analysis that, although it does not abolish the need to place arbitrary numerical values on life and limb, avoids the buck stopping with the unfortunate health economist. This approach, known as *cost–consequences analysis*, presents the results of the economic analysis in a disaggregated form. In other words, it expresses different outcomes in terms of their different natural units (i.e. something real such as months of survival, legs amputated or take-home babies), so that individuals can assign their own values to particular health states before comparing two quite different interventions (e.g. infertility treatment vs cholesterol lowering, as in the example I mentioned in Chapter 1). Cost–consequences analysis allows for the health state preference values of both individuals and society to change with time, and is particularly useful when these are disputed or likely to change. This approach may also allow the analysis to be used by different groups or societies from the ones on which the original trial was performed.

Ten questions to ask about an economic analysis

The elementary checklist that follows is based largely on the sources mentioned in the first paragraph of this chapter. I strongly recommend that for a more definitive list, you check out these sources – especially the official recommendations by the BMJ working group [1].

Question One: Is the analysis based on a study that answers a clearly defined clinical question about an economically important issue?

Before you attempt to digest what a paper says about costs, quality of life scales or utilities, make sure that the trial being analysed is scientifically relevant and capable of giving unbiased and unambiguous answers to the clinical question posed in its introduction (see Chapter 4). Furthermore, if there is clearly little to choose between the interventions in terms of either costs or benefits, a detailed economic analysis is probably pointless.

Question Two: Whose viewpoint are costs and benefits being considered from?
From the patient's point of view, he or she generally wants to get better as quickly as possible. From the Treasury's point of view, the most cost-effective health intervention is one that returns all citizens promptly to taxpayer status and, when this status is no longer tenable, causes immediate sudden death. From the drug company's point of view, it would be difficult to imagine a cost–benefit equation that did not contain one of the company's products, and from a physiotherapist's point of view, the removal of a physiotherapy service would never be cost-effective. There is no such thing as an economic analysis that is devoid of perspective. Most assume the perspective of the health care system itself, although some take into account the hidden costs to the patient and society (e.g. as a result of work days lost). There is no 'right' perspective for an economic evaluation – but the paper should say clearly whose costs and whose benefits have been counted 'in' and 'out'.

Question Three: Have the interventions being compared been shown to be clinically effective?
Nobody wants inexpensive treatment if it doesn't work. The paper you are reading may simply be an economic analysis, in which case it will be based on a previously published clinical trial, or it will be an economic evaluation of a new trial whose clinical results are presented in the same paper. Either way, you must make sure that the intervention that 'works out cheaper' is not substantially less effective in clinical terms than the one that stands to be rejected on the grounds of cost. (Note, however, that in a resource-limited health care system, it is often sensible to use treatments that are a little less effective when they are a lot less expensive than the best on offer!).

Question Four: Are the interventions sensible and workable in the settings where they are likely to be applied?
A research trial that compares one obscure and unaffordable intervention with another will have little impact on medical practice. Remember that standard current practice (which may be 'doing nothing') should almost certainly be one of the alternatives compared. Too many research trials look at intervention packages that would be impossible to implement in the non-research setting (e.g. they assume that general practitioners will own a state-of-the-art computer and agree to follow a protocol, that infinite nurse time is available for the taking of blood tests or that patients

will make their personal treatment choices solely on the basis of the trial's primary outcome measure).

Question Five: Which method of analysis was used, and was this appropriate?
This decision can be summarised as given here (see section 'How can we help ensure that evidence-based guidelines are followed?').

(a) If the interventions produced identical outcomes ⇒ cost-minimisation analysis.

(b) If the important outcome is unidimensional ⇒ cost-effectiveness analysis.

(c) If the important outcome is multi-dimensional ⇒ cost – utility analysis.

(d) If the outcomes can be expressed meaningfully in monetary terms (i.e. if it is possible to weigh the cost – benefit equation for this condition against the cost – benefit equation for another condition) ⇒ cost – benefit analysis.

(e) If a cost – benefit analysis would otherwise be appropriate but the preference values given to different health states are disputed or likely to change ⇒ cost – consequences analysis.

Question Six: How were costs and benefits measured?
Look back at section 'How can we help ensure that evidence-based guidelines are followed?', where I outlined some of the costs associated with my appendix operation. Now imagine a more complicated example – the rehabilitation of stroke patients into their own homes with attendance at a day centre compared with a standard alternative intervention (rehabilitation in a long-stay hospital). The economic analysis must take into account not just the time of the various professionals involved, the time of the secretaries and administrators who help run the service, and the cost of the food and drugs consumed by the stroke patients but also a fraction of the capital cost of building the day centre and maintaining a transport service to and from it.

There are no hard and fast rules for deciding which costs to include. If calculating 'cost per case' from first principles, remember that someone has to pay for heating, lighting, personnel support and even the accountants' bills of the institution. In general terms, these 'hidden costs' are known as overheads, and generally add an additional 30 – 60% onto the cost of a project. The task of costing things like operations and outpatient visits in the UK is easier than it used to be because these experiences are now bought and sold at a price that reflects (or should reflect) all overheads involved. Be warned, however, that unit costs of health interventions calculated in one country often bear no relation to those of the same intervention elsewhere, even when these costs are expressed as a proportion of GNP.

Benefits such as earlier return to work for a particular individual can, on the face of it, be measured in terms of the cost of employing that person at his or her usual daily rate. This approach has the unfortunate and politically unacceptable consequence of valuing the health of professional people higher than that of manual workers, homemakers or the unemployed, and that of the white majority higher than that of (generally) lower paid minority ethnic groups. It might therefore be preferable to derive the cost of sick days from the average national wage.

In a cost-effectiveness analysis, changes in health status will be expressed in natural units (see section 'How can we help ensure that evidence-based guidelines are followed?'). But just because the units are natural does not automatically make them appropriate. For example, the economic analysis of the treatment of peptic ulcer by two different drugs might measure outcome as 'proportion of ulcers healed after a 6-week course'. Treatments could be compared according to the cost per ulcer healed. However, if the relapse rates on the two drugs were very different, drug A might be falsely deemed 'more cost-effective' than drug B. A better outcome measure here might be 'ulcers which remained healed at one year'.

In cost–benefit analysis, where health status is expressed in utility units, such as QALYs, you would, if you were being really rigorous about evaluating the paper, look back at how the particular utilities used in the analysis were derived (see section 'How can we help ensure that evidence-based guidelines are followed?'). In particular, you will want to know whose health preference values were used – those of patients, doctors, health economists or the government.

Question Seven: Were incremental, rather than absolute, benefits considered?

This question is best illustrated by a simple example. Let's say drug X, at £100 per course, cures 10 out of every 20 patients. Its new competitor, drug Y, costs £120 per course and cures 11 out of 20 patients. The cost per case cured with drug X is £200 (because you spent £2000 curing 10 people), and the cost per case cured with drug Y is £218 (because you spent £2400 curing 11 people).

The *incremental* cost of drug Y – that is, the extra cost of curing the extra patient – is NOT £18 but £400, as this is the total amount extra that you have had to pay to achieve an outcome over and above what you would have achieved by giving all patients the cheaper drug. This striking example should be borne in mind the next time a pharmaceutical representative tries to persuade you that his or her product is 'more effective and only marginally more expensive'.

Question Eight: Was the 'here and now' given precedence over the distant future?

A bird in the hand is worth two in the bush. In health as well as money terms, we value a benefit today more highly than we value a promise of the same benefit in 5 years' time. When the costs or benefits of an intervention (or lack of the intervention) will occur sometime in the future, their value should be *discounted* to reflect this. The actual amount of discount that should be allowed for future, as opposed to immediate, health benefit, is pretty arbitrary, but most analyses use a figure of around 5% per year.

Question Nine: Was a sensitivity analysis performed?

Let's say a cost–benefit analysis comes out as saying that hernia repair by day-case surgery costs £1500 per QALY, whereas traditional open repair, with its associated hospital stay, costs £2100 per QALY. But, when you look at how the calculations were performed, you are surprised at how cheaply the laparoscopic equipment has been costed. If you raise the price of this equipment by 25%, does day-case surgery still come out dramatically cheaper? It may, or it may not.

Sensitivity analysis, or exploration of 'what-ifs', was described in section 'Validating diagnostic tests against a gold standard' in relation to meta-analysis. Exactly the same principles apply here: if adjusting the figures to account for the full range of possible influences gives you a totally different answer, you should not place too much reliance on the analysis. For a good example of a sensitivity analysis on a topic of both scientific and political importance, see this paper on the cost-effectiveness of statin therapy in people with different levels of baseline risk for cardiovascular disease [11].

Question Ten: Were "bottom line" aggregate scores overused?

In section 'How can we help ensure that evidence-based guidelines are followed?', I introduced the notion of cost–consequences analysis, in which the reader of the paper can attach his or her own values to different utilities. In practice, this is an unusual way of presenting an economic analysis, and, more commonly, the reader is faced with a cost–utility or cost–benefit analysis that gives a composite score in unfamiliar units which do not translate readily into exactly what gains and losses the patient can expect. The situation is analogous to the father who is told, 'your child's intelligence quotient is 115', when he would feel far better informed if he were presented with the disaggregated data: 'Johnny can read, write, count, and draw pretty well for his age'.

Conclusion

I hope this chapter has shown that the critical appraisal of an economic analysis rests as crucially on asking questions such as, 'where did those numbers come from?' and 'have any numbers been left out?' as on checking that the sums themselves were correct. Whilst few papers will fulfil all the criteria listed in section 'Ten questions to ask about an economic analysis' and summarised in Appendix 1, you should, after reading the chapter, be able to distinguish an economic analysis of moderate or good methodological quality from one which slips 'throwaway costings' ('drug X costs less than drug Y; therefore it is more cost-effective') into its results or discussion section.

References

1 Drummond M, Jefferson T. Guidelines for authors and peer reviewers of economic submissions to the BMJ. The BMJ Economic Evaluation Working Party. BMJ: British Medical Journal 1996;**313**(7052):275.
2 Jefferson T, Demicheli V, Mugford M. *Elementary economic evaluation in health care*. London: BMJ Books, 2000.
3 Donaldson C, Mitton C. *Priority setting toolkit: guide to the use of economics in healthcare decision making*. Oxford, John Wiley & Sons, 2009.
4 McDowell I, Newell C, McDowell I. *Measuring health: a guide to rating scales and questionnaires*. New York: Oxford University Press, 2006.
5 Bradley C, Speight J. Patient perceptions of diabetes and diabetes therapy: assessing quality of life. Diabetes/Metabolism Research and Reviews 2002;**18**(S3):S64–9.
6 Bache I. Measuring quality of life for public policy: an idea whose time has come? Agenda-setting dynamics in the European Union. Journal of European Public Policy 2013;**20**(1):21–38.
7 Fairclough DL. *Design and analysis of quality of life studies in clinical trials*. Boca Raton: CRC Press, 2010.
8 Phillips D. *Quality of life: concept, policy and practice*. Oxon: Routledge, 2012.
9 Young T, Yang Y, Brazier JE, et al. The first stage of developing preference-based measures: constructing a health-state classification using Rasch analysis. Quality of Life Research 2009;**18**(2):253–65.
10 Henderson C, Knapp M, Fernández J-L, et al. Cost effectiveness of telehealth for patients with long term conditions (Whole Systems Demonstrator telehealth questionnaire study): nested economic evaluation in a pragmatic, cluster randomised controlled trial. BMJ: British Medical Journal 2013;346:f1035.
11 Jha V, Modi GK. Cardiovascular disease: the price of a QALY – cost-effectiveness of statins in CKD. Nature Reviews Nephrology 2013;**9**:377–9.
12 Herman WH, Edelstein SL, Ratner RE, et al. The 10-year cost-effectiveness of lifestyle intervention or metformin for diabetes prevention: an intent-to-treat analysis of the DPP/DPPOS. Diabetes Care 2012;**35**(4):723–30.
13 Martin NK, Vickerman P, Miners A, et al. Cost-effectiveness of hepatitis C virus antiviral treatment for injection drug user populations. Hepatology 2012;**55**(1):49–57.
14 Saariniemi KM, Kuokkanen HO, Räsänen P, et al. The cost utility of reduction mammaplasty at medium-term follow-up: a prospective study. Journal of Plastic, Reconstructive & Aesthetic Surgery 2012;**65**(1):17–21.
15 Shahab L: *Cost-effectiveness of pharmacotherapy for smoking cessation*. London: National Centre for Smoking Cessation and Training (NCSCT), 2012 Available online http://www.ncsct.co.uk/usr/pub/B7_Cost-effectiveness _pharmacotherapy.pdf; accessed 5.11.13.

16 Coyle D, Coyle K, Cameron C, et al. Cost-effectiveness of new oral anticoagulants compared with warfarin in preventing stroke and other cardiovascular events in patients with atrial fibrillation. Value in Health 2013;**16**:498–506.
17 Frederix GW, Severens JL, Hövels AM, et al. Reviewing the cost-effectiveness of endocrine early breast cancer therapies: influence of differences in modeling methods on outcomes. Value in Health 2012;**15**(1):94–105.
18 Harris J. QALYfying the value of life. Journal of Medical Ethics 1987;**13**(3):117–23.
19 Whitehead SJ, Ali S. Health outcomes in economic evaluation: the QALY and utilities. British Medical Bulletin 2010;**96**(1):5–21.
20 Gold MR, Stevenson D, Fryback DG. HALYS and QALYS and DALYS, Oh My: similarities and differences in summary measures of population health. Annual Review of Public Health 2002;**23**(1):115–34.

Chapter 12   Papers that go beyond numbers (qualitative research)

What is qualitative research?

Twenty-five years ago, when I took up my first research post, a work-weary colleague advised me: 'Find something to measure, and keep on measuring it until you've got a boxful of data. Then stop measuring and start writing up'.

'But what should I measure?', I asked.

'That', he said cynically, 'doesn't much matter'.

This true example illustrates the limitations of an exclusively quantitative (counting-and-measuring) perspective in research. Epidemiologist Nick Black has argued that a finding or a result is more likely to be accepted as a fact if it is quantified (expressed in numbers) than if it is not [1]. There is little or no scientific evidence, for example, to support the well-known 'facts' that one couple in 10 is infertile or that one person in 10 is homosexual. Yet, observes Black, most of us are happy to accept uncritically such simplified, reductionist and blatantly incorrect statements so long as they contain at least one number.

Qualitative researchers seek a deeper truth. They aim to 'study things in their natural setting, attempting to make sense of, or interpret, phenomena in terms of the meanings people bring to them' [2], and they use 'a holistic perspective which preserves the complexities of human behaviour' [2].

Interpretive or qualitative research was for years the territory of the social scientists. It is now increasingly recognised as being not just complementary to but, in many cases, a prerequisite for the quantitative research with which most us who trained in the biomedical sciences are more familiar. Certainly, the view that the two approaches are mutually exclusive has itself become 'unscientific', and it is currently rather trendy, particularly in the fields of primary care and health services research, to say that you are doing some qualitative research – and since the first edition of this book was published,

How to Read a Paper: The Basics of Evidence-Based Medicine, Fifth Edition. Trisha Greenhalgh.
© 2014 John Wiley & Sons, Ltd. Published 2014 by John Wiley & Sons, Ltd.

qualitative research has even become mainstream within the evidence-based medicine movement [3, 4], and, as described in Chapter 7, there have been major developments in the science of integrating qualitative and quantitative evidence in the development and evaluation of complex interventions.

The late Dr Cecil Helman, an anthropologist as well as a medical doctor, told me the following story to illustrate the qualitative–quantitative dichotomy. A small child runs in from the garden and says, excitedly, 'Mummy, the leaves are falling off the trees'.

'Tell me more', says his mother.

'Well, five leaves fell in the first hour, then ten leaves fell in the second hour … '

That child will become a quantitative researcher.

A second child, when asked 'tell me more', might reply, 'Well, the leaves are big and flat, and mostly yellow or red, and they seem to be falling off some trees but not others. And mummy, why did no leaves fall last month?'

That child will become a qualitative researcher.

Questions such as 'How many parents would consult their general practitioner when their child has a mild temperature?', or 'What proportion of smokers have tried to give up?' clearly need answering through quantitative methods. But questions like 'Why do parents worry so much about their children's temperature?', and 'What stops people giving up smoking?' cannot and should not be answered by leaping in and measuring the first aspect of the problem that we (the outsiders) think might be important. Rather, we need to hang out, listen to what people have to say and explore the ideas and concerns that the individuals themselves come up with. After a while, we may notice a pattern emerging, which may prompt us to make our observations in a different way. We may start with one of the methods shown in Table 12.1, and go on to use a selection of others.

Box 12.1, which is reproduced with permission from Nick Mays and Catherine Pope's introductory paper 'Qualitative Research in Health Care' [5] summarises (indeed overstates) the differences between the qualitative and quantitative approaches to research. In reality, there is a great deal of overlap between them, the importance of which is increasingly being recognised [6].

As section 'Three preliminary questions to get your bearings' explains, quantitative research should begin with an idea (usually articulated as a hypothesis), which then, through measurement, generates data and, by *deduction*, allows a conclusion to be drawn. Qualitative research is different. It begins with an intention to explore a particular area, collects 'data' (e.g. observations, interviews, documents – even emails can count as qualitative data), and generates ideas and hypotheses from these data largely through what is known as *inductive reasoning* [2]. The strength of quantitative

Table 12.1 Examples of qualitative research methods

Ethnography (passive observation)	Systematic watching of behaviour and talk in natural occurring settings
Ethnography (participant observation)	Observation in which the researcher also occupies a role or part in the setting in addition to observing
Semi-structured interview	Face-to-face (or telephone) conversation with the purpose of exploring issues or topics in detail. Uses a broad list of questions or topics (known as a *topic guide*).
Narrative interview	Interview undertaken in a less structured fashion, with the purpose of getting a long story from the interviewee (typically a life story or the story of how an illness has unfolded over time). The interviewer holds back from prompting except to say 'tell me more'.
Focus groups	Method of group interview which explicitly includes and uses the group interaction to generate data
Discourse analysis	Detailed study of the words, phrases and formats used in particular social contexts (includes the study of naturally occurring talk as well as written materials such as policy documents or minutes of meetings)

Box 12.1 Qualitative versus quantitative research – the overstated dichotomy > (see reference [7])

	Qualitative	Quantitative
Social theory	Action	Structure
Methods	Observation, interview	Experiment, survey
Question	What is X? (classification)	How many Xs? (enumeration)
Reasoning	Inductive	Deductive
Sampling method	Theoretical	Statistical
Strength	Validity	Reliability

---

approach lies in its *reliability* (repeatability) – that is, the same measurements should yield the same results time after time. The strength of qualitative research lies in *validity* (closeness to the truth) – that is, good qualitative research, using a selection of data collection methods, really should touch the core of what is going on rather than just skimming the surface. The validity of qualitative methods is said to be greatly improved by the use of more than one method (see Table 12.1) in combination (a process sometimes known as *triangulation*), by the researcher thinking carefully about what is going on and how their own perspective might be influencing the data (an approach known as *reflexivity*) [7], and – some would argue – by more than one researcher analysing the same data independently (to demonstrate *inter-rater reliability*).

Since I wrote the first edition of this book, inter-rater reliability has become less credible as a measure of quality in qualitative research. Appraisers of qualitative papers increasingly seek to assess the competence and reflexivity of a single researcher rather than confirm that the findings were 'checked by someone else'. This change is attributable to two important insights. First, in most qualitative research, one person knows the data far better than anyone else, so the idea that two heads are better than one simply isn't true – a researcher who has been brought in merely to verify 'themes' may rely far more on personal preconceptions and guesswork than the main field worker. And second, with the trend towards more people from biomedical backgrounds doing qualitative research, it's not at all uncommon for two (or even a whole team of) naïve and untrained researchers setting up focus groups or attacking the free-text responses of questionnaires. Not only does 'agreement' between these individuals not correspond to quality but teams from similar backgrounds are also likely to bring similar biases, so high inter-rater reliability scores may be entirely spurious.

Those who are ignorant about qualitative research often believe that it constitutes little more than hanging out and watching leaves fall. It is beyond the scope of this book to take you through the substantial literature on how to (and how not to) proceed when observing, interviewing, leading a focus group, and so on. But sophisticated methods for all these techniques certainly exist, and if you are interested I suggest you try the excellent BMJ series by Scott Reeves and colleagues from Canada [8–12].

Qualitative methods really come into their own when researching uncharted territory – that is, where the variables of greatest concern are poorly understood, ill-defined and cannot be controlled. In such circumstances, the definitive hypothesis may not be arrived at until the study is well under way. But it is in precisely these circumstances that the qualitative researcher must ensure that he or she has, at the outset, carefully delineated a particular focus of research and identified some specific questions to try to answer (see Question One in section 'Evaluating papers that describe qualitative research'). The methods of qualitative research allow for – indeed, they require – modification of the research question in the light of findings generated along the way – a technique known as *progressive focusing* [5]. (In contrast, as 'd' of section 'Have the authors set the scene correctly?' showed, sneaking a look at the interim results of a quantitative study is statistically invalid!).

The so-called *iterative* approach (altering the research methods and the hypothesis as you go along) employed by qualitative researchers shows a commendable sensitivity to the richness and variability of the topic. Failure to recognise the legitimacy of this approach has, in the past, led critics to accuse qualitative researchers of continually moving their own goalposts. Whilst these criticisms are often misguided, there is a danger that when qualitative research is undertaken unrigorously by naïve researchers, the 'iterative' approach will slide into confusion. This is one reason why qualitative researchers must allow periods away from their fieldwork for reflection, planning and consultation with colleagues.

Evaluating papers that describe qualitative research

By its very nature, qualitative research is non-standard, unconfined and dependent on the subjective experience of both the researcher and the researched. It explores what needs to be explored and cuts its cloth accordingly. As implied in the previous section, qualitative research is an in-depth, interpretive task, not a technical procedure. It depends crucially on a competent and experienced researcher exercising the kind of skills and judgements that are difficult, if not impossible, to measure objectively. It is debatable, therefore, whether an all-encompassing critical appraisal checklist along the lines of the Users' Guides to the Medical Literature for quantitative research could ever be developed, although valiant attempts have been made [3, 4, 10, 13]. Some people have argued that critical appraisal checklists potentially detract from research quality in qualitative research because they encourage a mechanistic and protocol-driven approach [14].

My own view, and that of a number of individuals who have attempted, or are currently working on, this very task, is that such a checklist may not be as exhaustive or as universally applicable as the various guides for appraising quantitative research, but that it is certainly possible to set some ground rules. Without doubt, the best attempt to offer guidance (and also the best exposition of the uncertainties and unknowables) has been made by Dixon-Woods and her colleagues [15]. The list that follows has been distilled from the published work cited elsewhere in this chapter, and also from discussions many years ago with Dr Rod Taylor, who produced one of the earliest critical appraisal guides for qualitative papers.

Question One: Did the paper describe an important clinical problem addressed via a clearly formulated question?

In section 'Three preliminary questions to get your bearings', I explained that one of the first things you should look for in any research paper is a statement of why the research was carried out and what specific question it addressed. Qualitative papers are no exception to this rule: there is absolutely no scientific value in interviewing or observing people just for the sake of it. Papers which cannot define their topic of research more closely than 'we decided to interview 20 patients with epilepsy' inspire little confidence that the researchers really knew what they were studying or why.

You might be more inclined to read on if the paper stated in its introduction something like, 'Epilepsy is a common and potentially disabling condition, and a significant proportion of patients do not remain fit-free on medication. Antiepileptic medication is known to have unpleasant side effects, and several studies have shown that a high proportion of patients do not take their tablets regularly. We therefore decided to explore patients' beliefs about epilepsy and their perceived reasons for not taking their medication'. As I explained in section 'What is qualitative research?', the iterative nature of qualitative research is such that the definitive research question may not be clearly focused at the outset of the study, but it should certainly have been formulated by the time the report is written!

Question Two: Was a qualitative approach appropriate?

If the objective of the research was to explore, interpret or obtain a deeper understanding of a particular clinical issue, qualitative methods were almost certainly the most appropriate ones to use. If, however, the research aimed to achieve some other goal (such as determining the incidence of a disease or the frequency of an adverse drug reaction, testing a cause-and-effect hypothesis, or showing that one drug has a better risk–benefit ratio than another), qualitative methods are clearly inappropriate! If you think a case–control, cohort study or randomised trial would have been better suited to the research question posed in the paper than the qualitative methods that were actually used, you might like to compare that question with the examples in section 'Randomised controlled trials' to confirm your hunch.

Question Three: How were (a) the setting and (b) the subjects selected?

Look back at Box 12.1, which contrasts the *statistical* sampling methods of quantitative research with *theoretical* ones of qualitative research. Let me explain what this means. In the earlier chapters, particularly section 'Whom is the study about?', I emphasised the importance, in quantitative research, of ensuring that a truly random sample of participants is recruited. A random sample will ensure that the results reflect, on average, the condition of the population from which that sample was drawn.

In qualitative research, however, we are not interested in an 'on-average' view of a patient population. We want to gain an in-depth understanding of the experience of particular individuals or groups, and we should, therefore, deliberately seek out individuals or groups who fit the bill. If, for example, we wished to study the experience of women when they gave birth in hospital, we would be perfectly justified in going out of our way to find women who had had a range of different birth experiences – an induced delivery, an emergency Caesarean section, a delivery by a medical student, a late miscarriage, and so on.

We would also wish to select some women who had had shared antenatal care between an obstetrician and their general practitioner, and some women who had been cared for by community midwives throughout the pregnancy. In this example, it might be particularly instructive to find women who had had their care provided by male doctors, even though this would be a relatively unusual situation. Finally, we might choose to study patients who gave birth in the setting of a large, modern, 'high-tech' maternity unit as well as some who did so in a small community hospital. Of course, all these specifications will give us 'biased' samples, but that is exactly what we want.

Watch out for qualitative research where the sample has been selected (or appears to have been selected) purely on the basis of convenience. In the above-mentioned example, taking the first dozen patients to pass through the nearest labour ward would be the easiest way to notch up interviews, but the information obtained may be considerably less helpful.

Question Four: What was the researcher's perspective, and has this been taken into account?

Given that qualitative research is necessarily grounded in real-life experience, a paper describing such research should not be 'trashed' simply because the researchers have declared a particular cultural perspective or personal involvement with the participants of the research. Quite the reverse: they should be congratulated for doing just that. It is important to recognise that there is no way of abolishing, or fully controlling for, observer bias in qualitative research. This is most obviously the case when participant observation (see Table 12.1) is used, but it is also true for other forms of data collection and of data analysis.

If, for example, the research concerns the experience of adults with asthma living in damp and overcrowded housing and the perceived effect of these surroundings on their health, the data generated by techniques such as focus groups or semi-structured interviews are likely to be heavily influenced by what the *interviewer* believes about this subject and by whether he or she is employed by the hospital chest clinic, the social work department of the local authority, or an environmental pressure group. But because it is inconceivable that the interviews could have been conducted by someone with no views at all and no ideological or cultural perspective, the most that can be required of the researchers is that they describe in detail where they are coming from so that the results can be interpreted accordingly.

It is for this reason, incidentally, that qualitative researchers generally prefer to write up their work in the first person ('I interviewed the participants' rather than 'the participants were interviewed'), because this makes explicit the role and influence of the researcher.

Question Five: What methods did the researcher use for collecting data – and are these described in enough detail?

I once spent 2 years doing highly quantitative, laboratory-based experimental research in which around 15 h of every week were spent filling or emptying test tubes. There was a standard way to fill the test tubes, a standard way to spin them in the centrifuge, and even a standard way to wash them up. When I finally published my research, some 900 h of drudgery was summed up in a single sentence: 'Patients' serum rhubarb levels were measured according to the method described by Bloggs and Bloggs [reference to Bloggs and Bloggs' paper on how to measure serum rhubarb]'.

I now spend quite a lot of my time doing qualitative research, and I can confirm that it's infinitely more fun. My research colleagues and I have spent some 15 years exploring the beliefs, hopes, fears and attitudes of diabetic patients from the minority ethnic groups in the East End of London (we began with British Bangladeshis and extended the work to other South Asian and – later – other ethnic groups). We had to develop, for example, a valid way of simultaneously translating and transcribing interviews that were conducted in Sylheti, a complex dialect of Bengali which has no written form. We found that participants' attitudes appear to be heavily influenced by the presence in the room of certain of their relatives, so we contrived to interview some patients in both the presence and the absence of these key relatives.

I could go on describing the methods we devised to address this particular research topic, but I have probably made my point: the methods section of a qualitative paper often cannot be written in shorthand or dismissed by reference to someone else's research techniques. It may have to be lengthy and discursive because it is telling a unique story without which the results cannot be interpreted. As with the sampling strategy, there are no hard and fast rules about exactly what details should be included in this section of the paper. You should simply ask, 'have I been given enough information about the methods used?', and, if you have, use your common sense to assess, 'are these methods a sensible and adequate way of addressing the research question?'

Question Six: What methods did the researcher use to analyse the data – and what quality control measures were implemented?

The data analysis section of a qualitative research paper is the opportunity for the researcher(s) to demonstrate the difference between sense and non-sense. Having amassed a thick pile of completed interview transcripts or field notes, the genuine qualitative researcher has hardly begun. It is simply not good enough to flick through the text looking for 'interesting quotes' to support a particular theory. The researcher must find a *systematic* way of analysing his or her data, and, in particular, must seek to detect and interpret items of data that appear to contradict or challenge the theories derived from the majority. One of the best short articles on qualitative data analysis was published by Cathy Pope and Sue Ziebland in the *British Medical Journal* a few years ago – look it out if you're new to this field and want to know where to start [16]. If you want the definitive textbook on qualitative research, which describes multiple different approaches to analysis, try the marvellous tome edited by Denzin and Lincoln [2].

By far the commonest way of analysing the kind of qualitative data that is generally collected in biomedical research is *thematic analysis*. In this, the researchers go through printouts of free text, draw up a list of broad themes and allocate coding categories to each. For example, a 'theme' might be patients' knowledge about their illness and within this theme, codes might include 'transmissible causes', 'supernatural causes', 'causes due to own behaviour', and so on. Note that these codes do not correspond to a conventional biomedical taxonomy ('genetic', 'infectious', 'metabolic', and so on), because the point of the research is to explore the interviewees' taxonomy, whether the researcher agrees with it or not. Thematic analysis is often tackled by drawing up a matrix or framework with a new column for each theme and a new row for each 'case' (e.g. an interview transcript), and cutting and pasting relevant segments of text into each box [13]. Another type of thematic analysis is the constant comparative method – in which each new piece of data is compared with the emerging summary of all the previous items, allowing step-by-step refinement of an emerging theory [17].

Quite commonly these days, qualitative data analysis is performed with the help of a computer programme such as ATLAS-TI or NVIVO, which makes it much easier to handle large datasets. The statements made by all the interviewees on a particular topic can be compared with one another, and sophisticated comparisons can be made such as 'did people who made statement A also tend to make statement B?' But remember, a qualitative computer programme does not analyse the data by autopilot, any more than a quantitative programme like SPSS can tell the researcher which statistical test to apply in each case! Whilst the sentence 'data were analysed using NVIVO' might appear impressive, the GIGO rule (garbage in, garbage out) often applies. Excellent qualitative data analysis can occur using the VLDRT (very large dining room table) method, in which printouts of (say) interviews are marked up with felt pens and (say) the constant comparative method is undertaken manually instead of electronically.

It's often difficult when writing up qualitative research to demonstrate how quality control was achieved. As mentioned in the previous section, just because the data have been analysed by more than one researcher does not *necessarily* assure rigour. Indeed, researchers who never disagree on their subjective judgements (is a particular paragraph in a patient's account really evidence of 'anxiety' or 'disempowerment' or 'trust'?) are probably not thinking hard enough about their own interpretations. The essence of quality in such circumstances is more to do with the level of critical dialogue between the researchers, and in *how* disagreements were exposed and resolved. In analysing my early research data on the health beliefs of British Bangladeshis with diabetes, for example, three of us looked in turn at a typed interview transcript and assigned codings to particular statements [18]. We then compared our decisions and argued (sometimes heatedly) about our disagreements. Our analysis revealed differences in the interpretation of certain statements that we were unable to fully resolve. For example, we never reached agreement about what the term *exercise* means in this ethnic group. This did not mean that one of us was 'wrong' but that there were *inherent* ambiguities in the data. Perhaps, for example, this sample of interviewees were themselves confused about what the term *exercise* means and the benefits it offers to people with diabetes.

Question Seven: Are the results credible, and if so, are they clinically important?
We obviously cannot assess the credibility of qualitative results via the precision and accuracy of measuring devices, nor their significance via confidence intervals and numbers needed to treat. The most important tool to determine whether the results are sensible and believable, and whether they matter in practice, is plain common sense.

One important aspect of the results section to check is whether the authors cite actual data. Claims such as 'general practitioners did not usually recognise the value of annual appraisal' would be more credible if one or two verbatim quotes from the interviewees were reproduced to illustrate them. The results should be independently and objectively verifiable (e.g. by including longer segments of text in an appendix or online resource), and all quotes and examples should be indexed so that they can be traced back to an identifiable interviewee and data source.

Question Eight: What conclusions were drawn, and are they justified by the results?

A quantitative research paper, presented in standard Introduction, Methods, Research and Discussion (IMRAD) format (see section 'The science of "trashing" papers'), should clearly distinguish the study's results (usually a set of numbers) from the interpretation of those results. The reader should have no difficulty separating what the researchers *found* from what they think it *means*. In qualitative research, however, such a distinction is rarely possible, as the results are by definition an interpretation of the data. It is therefore necessary, when assessing the validity of qualitative research, to ask whether the interpretation placed on the data accords with common sense and that the researcher's personal, professional and cultural perspective is made explicit so the reader can assess the 'lens' through which the researcher has undertaken the fieldwork, analysis and interpretation. This can be a difficult exercise because the language we use to describe things tends to impugn meanings and motives that the participants themselves may not share. Compare, for example, the two statements, 'three women went to the well to get water' and 'three women met at the well and each was carrying a pitcher'.

It is becoming a cliché that the conclusions of qualitative studies, like those of all research, should be 'grounded in evidence' – that is, that they should flow from what the researchers found in the field. Mays and Pope [5] suggest three useful questions for determining whether the conclusions of a qualitative study are valid.

• How well does this analysis explain why people behave in the way they do?
• How comprehensible would this explanation be to a thoughtful participant in the setting?
• How well does the explanation cohere with what we already know?

Question Nine: Are the findings of the study transferable to other settings?

One of the commonest criticisms of qualitative research is that the findings of any qualitative study pertain only to the limited setting in which they were obtained. In fact, this is not necessarily any truer of qualitative research than of quantitative research. Look back at the example of women's birth experiences that I described in Question Three. A convenience sample of the first dozen women to give birth would provide little more than the collected experiences of these 12 women. A *purposive* sample as described in Question Three would extend the transferability of the findings to women having a wide range of birth experience. But by making iterative adjustments to the sampling frame as the research study unfolds, the researchers will be able to develop a theoretical sample and test new theories as they emerge. For example (and note, I'm making this example up), the researchers might find that better educated women seem to have more psychologically traumatic experiences than less well educated women. This might lead to a new hypothesis about women's expectations (the better educated the woman, the more she expects a 'perfect birth experience'), which would in turn lead to a change in the purposive sampling strategy (we now want to find extremes of maternal education), and so on. The more the research has been driven by this kind of progressive focusing and iterative data analysis, the more its findings are likely to be transferable beyond the sample itself.

Conclusion

Doctors have traditionally placed high value on number-based data, which may in reality be misleading, reductionist and irrelevant to the real issues. The increasing popularity of qualitative research in the biomedical sciences has arisen largely because quantitative methods provided either no answers, or the wrong answers, to important questions in both clinical care and service delivery. If you still feel that qualitative research is necessarily second rate by virtue of being a 'soft' science, you should be aware that you are out of step with the evidence.

In 1993, Catherine Pope and Nicky Britten presented at a conference a paper entitled 'Barriers to qualitative methods in the medical mindset', in which they showed their collection of rejection letters from biomedical journals [19]. The letters revealed a striking ignorance of qualitative methodology on the part of reviewers. In other words, the people who had rejected the papers often appeared to be incapable of distinguishing good qualitative research from bad.

Somewhat ironically, poor-quality qualitative papers now appear regularly in some medical journals, which appear to have undergone an about-face in editorial policy since Pope and Britten's exposure of the 'medical mindset'. I hope, therefore, that the questions listed earlier, and the subsequent references, will assist reviewers in both camps: those who continue to reject qualitative papers for the wrong reasons and those who have climbed on the qualitative bandwagon and are now *accepting* such papers for the wrong reasons! Note, however, that the critical appraisal of qualitative research is a relatively underdeveloped science, and the questions posed in this chapter are still being refined.

References

1 Black N. Why we need qualitative research. Journal of Epidemiology and Community Health 1994;**48**(5):425–6.
2 Denzin NK, Lincoln YS. *The SAGE handbook of qualitative research*. Sage, London, 2011.
3 Giacomini MK, Cook DJ. Users' guides to the medical literature XXIII. Qualitative research in health care A. Are the results of the study valid?. JAMA: The Journal of the American Medical Association 2000;**284**(3):357–62.
4 Giacomini MK, Cook D. Users' guides to the medical literature: XXIII. Qualitative research in health care B. What are the results and how do they help me care for my patients?. JAMA: The Journal of the American Medical Association 2000;**284**:478–82.
5 Mays N, Pope C. Qualitative research in health care: assessing quality in qualitative research. BMJ: British Medical Journal 2000;**320**(7226):50.
6 Dixon-Woods M, Agarwal S, Young B, et al. *Integrative approaches to qualitative and quantitative evidence*. London, Health Development Agency, 2004.
7 Gilgun JF. Reflexivity and qualitative research. Current Issues in Qualitative Research 2010;**1**(2):1–8.
8 Reeves S, Albert M, Kuper A, et al. Qualitative research: why use theories in qualitative research? BMJ: British Medical Journal 2008;**337**(7670):631–4.
9 Lingard L, Albert M, Levinson W. Grounded theory, mixed methods, and action research. BMJ: British Medical Journal 2008;**337**(aug07_3):a567–a67.
10 Kuper A, Lingard L, Levinson W. Critically appraising qualitative research. British Medical Journal 2008;**337**:a1035.
11 Kuper A, Reeves S, Levinson W. Qualitative research: an introduction to reading and appraising qualitative research. BMJ: British Medical Journal 2008; **337**(7666):404–7.
12 Reeves S, Kuper A, Hodges BD. Qualitative research methodologies: ethnography. BMJ: British Medical Journal 2008;**337**:a1020.
13 Spencer L, Britain G. *Quality in qualitative evaluation: a framework for assessing research evidence*. Government Chief Social Researcher's Office, Cabinet Office, London, 2003.
14 Barbour RS. Checklists for improving rigour in qualitative research a case of the tail wagging the dog? BMJ: British Medical Journal 2001;**322**(7294):1115.
15 Dixon-Woods M, Shaw RL, Agarwal S, et al. The problem of appraising qualitative research. Quality and Safety in Health Care 2004;**13**(3):223–5.
16 Pope C, Ziebland S, Mays N. Qualitative research in health care: analysing qualitative data. BMJ: British Medical Journal 2000;**320**(7227):114.
17 Glaser BG. The constant comparative method of qualitative analysis. Social Problems 1965;**12**(4):436–45.

18 Greenhalgh T, Helman C, Chowdhury AM. Health beliefs and folk models of diabetes in British Bangladeshis: a qualitative study. BMJ: British Medical Journal 1998;**316**(7136):978–83.
19 Pope C, Britten N. The quality of rejection: barriers to qualitative methods in the medical mindset. Paper presented at BSA Medical Sociology Group annual conference, 1993.

Chapter 13   **Papers that report questionnaire research**

The rise and rise of questionnaire research

When and where did you last fill out a questionnaire? They come through the door, and appear in our pigeon holes at work. We get them as email attachments and find them in the dentist's waiting room. The kids bring them home from school, and it's not uncommon for one to accompany the bill in a restaurant. I recently met someone at a party who described himself as a 'questionnaire mugger' – his job was to stop people in the street and take down their answers to a list of questions about their income, tastes, shopping preferences and goodness knows what else.

This chapter is based on a series of papers I edited for the *British Medical Journal*, written by a team led by my colleague Boynton [1–3]. Petra has taught me a great deal about this widely used research technique, including the fact that there's probably more bad questionnaire research in the literature than just about any other study design. While you need a laboratory to do bad lab work, and a supply of medicines to do bad pharmaceutical research, all you need to do to produce bad questionnaire research is write out a list of questions, photocopy it and ask a few people to fill it in. It's therefore somewhat odd that the otherwise very comprehensive Users' Guides to the Medical Literature published in the *Journal of the American Medical Association* do not (to my knowledge) include a paper on questionnaire studies.

Questionnaires are often considered as an 'objective' means of collecting information about people's knowledge, beliefs, attitudes and behaviour [4, 5]. Do our patients like our opening hours? What do teenagers think of a local anti-drugs campaign – and has it changed their attitudes? How much do nurses know about the management of asthma? What proportion of the population view themselves as gay or bisexual? Why don't doctors use computers to their maximum potential? You can probably see from these

---

How to Read a Paper: The Basics of Evidence-Based Medicine, Fifth Edition. Trisha Greenhalgh.
© 2014 John Wiley & Sons, Ltd. Published 2014 by John Wiley & Sons, Ltd.

examples that questionnaires can seek both quantitative data (*x* percent of people like our services) and qualitative data (people using our services have *xyz* experiences). In other words, questionnaires are not a 'quantitative method' or a 'qualitative method' but a tool for collecting a range of different types of data, depending on the question asked in each item and the format in which responders are expected to answer them.

I've already used the expression GIGO (garbage in, garbage out) in previous chapters to make the point that poorly structured instruments lead to poor quality data, misleading conclusions and woolly recommendations. Nowhere is that more true than in questionnaire research. While clear guidance on the design and reporting of randomised controlled trials (RCTs) and systematic reviews is now widely available (see the discussion about the CONSORT checklist in Chapter 6 and the QUORUM and PRISMA checklists in Chapter 9), there is no comparable framework for questionnaire research, although I'm told there is one being developed. Perhaps for this reason, despite a wealth of detailed guidance in the specialist literature [4, 5], elementary methodological errors are common in questionnaire research undertaken by health professionals [1–3].

Before we turn to the critical appraisal, a word about terminology. A questionnaire is a form of psychometric instrument – that is, it is designed to measure formally an aspect of human psychology. We sometimes refer to questionnaires as 'instruments'. The questions within a questionnaire are sometimes known as *items*. An item is the smallest unit within the questionnaire that is individually scored. It might comprise a stem ('pick which of the following responses corresponds to your own view') and then five possible options. Or it might be a simple 'yes/no' or 'true/false' response.

Ten questions to ask about a paper describing a questionnaire study

Question One: What was the research question, and was the questionnaire appropriate for answering it?
Look back to section 'The science of "trashing" papers', where I describe three preliminary questions to get you started in appraising any paper. The first of these was 'what was the research question – and why was the study needed?'. This is a particularly good starter question for questionnaire studies, because (as explained in the previous section) inexperienced researchers often embark on questionnaire research without clarifying why they are doing it or what they want to find out. In addition, people often decide to use a questionnaire for studies that need a totally different

method. Sometimes, a questionnaire will be appropriate but only if used within a mixed methodology study (e.g. to extend and quantify the findings of an initial exploratory phase). Table 13.1 gives some real examples based on papers that Petra Boynton and I collected from the published literature and offered by participants in courses we have run.

There are many advantages to researchers of using a previously validated and published questionnaire. The research team will save time and resources; they will be able to compare their own findings with those from other studies; they need only give outline details of the instrument when they write up their work; and they will not need to have gone through a thorough validation process for the instrument. Sadly, inexperienced researchers (most typically, students doing a dissertation) tend to forget to look thoroughly in the literature for a suitable 'off the peg' instrument, and such individuals often do not know about formal validation techniques (see subsequent text). Even though most such studies will be rejected by journal editors, a worrying proportion find their way into the literature.

Increasingly, health services research uses standard 'off the peg' questionnaires designed explicitly for producing data that can be compared across studies. For example, clinical trials routinely include standard instruments to measure patients' knowledge about a disease [6]; satisfaction with services [7]; or health-related quality of life (QoL) [8, 9]. The validity (see subsequent text) of this approach depends crucially on whether the type and range of closed responses (i.e. the list of possible answers that people are asked to select from) reflects the full range of perceptions and feelings that people in all the different potential sampling frames might actually hold.

Question Two: Was the questionnaire used in the study valid and reliable?
A valid questionnaire measures what it claims to measure. In reality, many fail to do this. For example, a self-completion questionnaire that seeks to measure people's food intake may be invalid, because in reality it measures what they *say* they have eaten, not what they have *actually* eaten [10]. Similarly, questionnaires asking general practitioners (GPs) how they manage particular clinical conditions have been shown to differ significantly from actual clinical practice [11]. Note that an instrument developed in a different time, country or cultural context may not be a valid measure in the group you are studying. Here's a quirky example. The item 'I often attend gay parties' was a valid measure of a person's sociability level in the UK in the 1950s, but the wording has a very different connotation today [1]! If you are interested in the measurement of QoL through questionnaires, you might like to look out for the controversy about the validity of such instruments when used beyond the context in which they were developed [12].

Table 13.1 Examples of research questions for which a questionnaire may *not* be the most appropriate design

Broad area of research	Example of research questions	Why is a questionnaire NOT the most appropriate method?	What method(s) should be used instead?
Burden of disease	What is the prevalence of asthma in schoolchildren?	A child may have asthma but the parent does not know it; parents may think incorrectly that their child has asthma; or they may withhold information that is perceived as stigmatising	Cross-sectional survey using standardised diagnostic criteria and/or systematic analysis of medical records
Professional behaviour	How do general practitioners manage low back pain?	What doctors say they do is not the same as what they actually do, especially when they think their practice is being judged by others	Direct observation or video recording of consultations; use of simulated patients; systematic analysis of medical records
Health-related lifestyle	What proportion of people in smoking cessation studies quit successfully?	The proportion of true quitters is less than the proportion who say they have quit. A similar pattern is seen in studies of dietary choices, exercise and other lifestyle factors	'Gold standard' diagnostic test (in this example, urinary or salivary cotinine)
Needs assessment in 'special needs' groups	What are the unmet needs of refugees and asylum seekers for health and social care services?	A questionnaire is likely to reflect the preconceptions of researchers (e.g. it may take existing services and/or the needs of more 'visible' groups as its starting point) and fail to tap into important areas of need	Range of exploratory qualitative methods designed to build up a 'rich picture' of the problem – for example, semi-structured interviews of users, health professionals and the voluntary sector; focus groups; and in-depth studies of critical events

Reliable questionnaires yield consistent results from repeated samples and different researchers over time [4, 5]. Differences in the results obtained from a reliable questionnaire come from differences between participants, and not from inconsistencies in how the items are understood or how different observers interpret the responses. A standardised questionnaire is one that is written and administered in a strictly set manner, so all participants are asked precisely the same questions in an identical format and responses recorded in a uniform manner. Standardising a measure increases its reliability. If you participated in the UK Census (General Household Survey) in 2011, you may remember being asked a rather mechanical set of questions. This is because the interviewer had been trained to administer the instrument in a highly standardised way, so as to increase reliability. It's often difficult to ascertain from a published paper how hard the researchers tried to achieve standardisation, but they may have quoted inter-rater reliability figures.

Question Three: What did the questionnaire look like, and was this appropriate for the target population?

When I say 'what did it look like?' I am talking about two things – form and content. Form concerns issues such as how many pages was it, was it visually appealing (or off-putting), how long did it take to fill in, the terminology used, and so on. These are not minor issues! A questionnaire that goes on for 30 pages, includes reams of scientific jargon, and contains questions that a respondent might find offensive, will not be properly filled in – and hence the results of a survey will be meaningless [2].

Content is about the actual items. Did the questions make sense, and could the participants in the sample understand them? Were any questions ambiguous or overly complicated? Were ambiguous weasel words such as 'frequently', 'regularly', 'commonly', 'usually', 'many', 'some' and 'hardly ever' avoided? Were the items 'open' (respondents can write anything they like) or 'closed' (respondents must pick from a list of options) – and if the latter, were all potential responses represented? Closed-ended designs enable researchers to produce aggregated data quickly, but the range of possible answers is set by the researchers, not the respondents, and the richness of responses is therefore much lower [13]. Some respondents (known as *yea-sayers*) tend to agree with statements rather than disagree. For this reason, researchers should not present their items so that 'strongly agree' always links to the same broad attitude. For example, on a patient satisfaction scale, if one question is 'my GP generally tries to help me out', another question should be phrased in the negative – for example, 'the receptionists are usually *impolite*'.

Question Four: Were the instructions clear?

If you have ever been asked to fill out a questionnaire and 'got lost' halfway through (or discovered you don't know where to send it once you've filled it in), you will know that instructions contribute crucially to the validity of the instrument. These include

- an explanation of what the study is about and what the overall purpose of the research is;
- an assurance of anonymity and confidentiality, as well as confirmation that the person can stop completing the questionnaire at any time without having to give a reason;
- clear and accurate contact details of whom to approach for further information;
- instructions on what they need to send back and a stamped addressed envelope if it is a postal questionnaire;
- adequate instructions on how to complete each item, with examples where necessary;
- any insert (e.g. leaflet), gift (e.g. book token) or honorarium, if these are part of the protocol.

These aspects of the study are unlikely to be listed in the published paper, but they may be in an appendix, and, if not, you should be able to get the information from the authors.

Question Five: Was the questionnaire adequately piloted?

Questionnaires often fail because participants don't understand them, can't complete them, get bored or offended by them or dislike how they look. Although friends and colleagues can help check spelling, grammar and layout, they cannot reliably predict the emotional reactions or comprehension difficulties of other groups. For this reason, all questionnaires (whether newly developed or 'off the peg') should be piloted on participants who are representative of the definitive study sample to see, for example, how long people take to complete the instrument, whether any items are misunderstood, or whether people get bored or confused halfway through. Three specific questions to ask are (i) What were the characteristics of the participants on whom the instrument was piloted; (ii) *How* was the piloting exercise undertaken – what details are given? and (iii) *In what ways* was the definitive instrument changed as a result of piloting?

Question Six: What was the sample?

If you have read the previous chapters, you will know that a skewed or non-representative sample will lead to misleading results and unsafe conclusions. When you appraise a questionnaire study, it's important to ask what the sampling frame was for the definitive study (purposive, random and snowball) and also whether it was sufficiently large and representative. Given here are the main types of sample for a questionnaire study (Table 13.2).

- *Random sample*: A target group is identified, and a random selection of people from that group is invited to participate. For example, a computer might be used to select a random one in four sample from a diabetes register.
- *Stratified random sample*: As random sample but the target group is first stratified according to a particular characteristic(s) – for example, diabetic people on insulin, tablets and diet. Random sampling is carried out separately for these different subgroups.
- *Snowball sample*: A small group of participants is identified and then asked to 'invite a friend' to complete the questionnaire. This group is in turn invited to nominate someone else, and so on.
- *Opportunity*: Usually for pragmatic reasons, the first people to appear who meet the criteria are asked to complete the questionnaire. This might happen, for example, in a busy GP surgery when all patients attending on a particular day are asked to fill out a survey about the convenience of opening hours. But such a sample is clearly biased, as those who find the opening hours inconvenient won't be there in the first place! This example should remind you that opportunity (sometimes known as *convenience*) samples are rarely if ever scientifically justified.
- *Systematically skewed sample*: Let's say you want to assess how satisfied patients are with their GP, and you already know from your pilot study that 80% of people from affluent postcodes will complete the questionnaire but only 60% of those from deprived postcodes will. You could oversample from the latter group to ensure that your dataset reflects the socio-economic make-up of your practice population. (Ideally, if you did this, you would also have to show that people who refused to fill out the questionnaire did not differ in key characteristics from those who completed it).

It is also important to consider whether the instrument was suitable for all participants and potential participants. In particular, did it take account of the likely range in the sample of physical and intellectual abilities, language and literacy, understanding of numbers or scaling and perceived threat of questions or questioner?

Question Seven: How was the questionnaire administered – and was the response rate adequate?

The methods section of a paper describing a questionnaire study should include details of three aspects of administration: (i) How was the questionnaire distributed (e.g. by post, face to face or electronically)? (ii) How was the questionnaire completed (e.g. self-completion or researcher-assisted)?

Table 13.2 Types of sampling frame for questionnaire research

Sample type	How it works	When to use
Opportunity/ haphazard	Participants are selected from a group who are available at time of study (e.g. patients attending a GP surgery on a particular morning)	Should be avoided if possible
Random	A target group is identified, and a random selection of people from that group is invited to participate. For example, a computer might be used to select a random one in four sample from a diabetes register	Use in studies where you wish to reflect the average viewpoint of a population
Stratified random	As random sample but the target group is first stratified according to a particular characteristic(s) – for example, diabetic people on insulin, tablets and diet. Random sampling is carried out separately for these different subgroups	Use when the target group is likely to have systematic differences by subgroup
Quota	Participants who match the wider population are identified (e.g. into groups such as social class, gender age, etc.). Researchers are given a set number within each group to interview (e.g. so many young middle-class women)	For studies where you want to reflect outcomes as closely representative of the wider population as possible. Frequently used in political opinion polls, and so on
Snowball	Participants are recruited, and asked to identify other similar people to take part in the research	Helpful when working with hard-to-reach groups (e.g. lesbian mothers)

and (iii) Were the response rates reported fully, including details of participants who were unsuitable for the research or refused to take part? Have any potential response biases been discussed?

The *British Medical Journal* will not usually publish a paper describing a questionnaire survey if fewer than 70% of people approached completed the questionnaire properly. There have been a number of research studies on how to increase the response rate to a questionnaire study. In summary, the following have all been shown to increase response rates [3].

- The questionnaire is clearly designed and has a simple layout.
- It offers participants incentives or prizes in return for completion.
- It has been thoroughly piloted and tested.
- Participants are notified about the study in advance, with a personalised invitation.
- The aim of the study and means of completing the questionnaire are clearly explained.
- A researcher is on hand to answer questions, and collect the completed questionnaire.
- If using a postal questionnaire, a stamped addressed envelope is included.
- The participants feel they are stakeholders in the study.
- Questions are phrased in a way that holds the participants' attention.
- The questionnaire has clear focus and purpose, and is kept concise.
- The questionnaire is appealing to look at.

Another thing to look for in relation to response rates is a table in the paper comparing the characteristics of people who responded with people who were approached but refused to fill out the questionnaire. If there were systematic (as opposed to chance) differences between these groups, the results of the survey will not be generalisable to the population from which the responders were drawn. Responders to surveys conducted in the street, for example, are often older than average (perhaps because they are in less of a hurry!), and less likely to be from an ethnic minority (perhaps because some of the latter are unable to speak the language of the researcher fluently). On the other hand, if the authors of the study have shown that non-responders are pretty similar to responders, you should worry less about generalisablity even if response rates were lower than you'd have liked.

Question Eight: How were the data analysed?

Analysis of questionnaire data is a sophisticated science. See these excellent textbooks on social research methods if you're interested in learning the formal techniques [4, 5]. If you are just interested in completing a checklist about a published questionnaire study, try considering these aspects of the study. First, broadly what sort of analysis was carried out and was this appropriate? In particular, were the correct statistical tests used for quantitative responses, and/or was a recognisable method of qualitative analysis (see section 'Measuring costs and benefits of health interventions') used for open-ended questions? It is reassuring (but by no means a flawless test) to learn that one of the paper's authors is a statistician. And as I said in Chapter 5, if the statistical tests used are ones you have never heard of, you should probably smell a rat. The vast majority of questionnaire data can be analysed using commonly used statistical tests such as Chi squared, Spearman's, Pearson correlation, and so on. The commonest mistake of all in questionnaire research is to use no statistical tests at all, and you don't need a PhD in statistics to spot that dodge!

You should also check to ensure that there is no evidence of 'data dredging'. In other words, have the authors simply thrown their data into a computer and run hundreds of tests, and then dreamt up a plausible hypothesis to go with something that comes out as 'significant'? In the jargon, all analyses should be hypothesis driven – that is, the hypothesis should be thought up first and then the analysis should be performed, not vice versa.

Question Nine: What were the main results?

Consider first what the overall findings were, and whether all relevant data were reported. Are quantitative results definitive (statistically significant), and are relevant *non-significant* results also reported? It may be just as important to have discovered, for example, that GPs' self-reported confidence in managing diabetes is *not* correlated to their knowledge about the condition as it would have been to discover that there was a correlation! For this reason, the questionnaire study that only comments on the 'positive' statistical associations is internally biased.

Another important question is have qualitative results been adequately interpreted (e.g. using an explicit theoretical framework), and have any quotes been properly justified and contextualised (rather than 'cherry picked' to spice up the paper)? Look back at Chapter 6 ('Papers that report drug trials and other simple interventions') and remind yourself of the tricks used by unscrupulous marketing people to oversell findings. Check carefully the graphs (especially the zero-intercept on axes) and the data tables.

Question Ten: What are the key conclusions?

This is a common-sense question. What do the results actually mean, and have the researchers drawn an appropriate link between the data and their conclusions? Have the findings been placed within the wider body of knowledge in the field (especially any similar or contrasting surveys using the same instrument)? Have the authors acknowledged the limitations of their study and couched their discussion in the light of these (e.g. if the sample was small or the response rate low, did they recommend further studies to confirm the preliminary findings)? Finally, are any recommendations fully justified by the findings? For example, if they have performed a small, parochial study they should not be suggesting changes in national policy as a result! If you are new to critical appraisal you may find such judgements difficult to make, and the best way to get better is to join in journal club discussions (either face to face or online) where a group of you share your common-sense reactions to a chosen paper.

In conclusion, anyone can write down a list of questions and photocopy it – but this doesn't mean that a set of responses to these questions constitutes research! The development, administration, analysis and reporting of questionnaire studies is at least as challenging as the other research approaches described in other chapters in this book. Questionnaire researchers are a disparate bunch, and have not yet agreed on a structured reporting format comparable to CONSORT (RCTs), QUORUM or PRISMA (systematic reviews) and AGREE (guidelines). Whilst a number of suggested structured tools, each designed for slightly different purposes, are now available [14–16], a review of such tools found little consensus and many unanswered questions [17]. I suspect that as such guides come to be standardised and more widely used, papers describing questionnaire research will be more consistent and easier to appraise.

References

1 Boynton PM, Wood GW, Greenhalgh T. A hands on guide to questionnaire research part three: reaching beyond the white middle classes. BMJ: British Medical Journal 2004;**328**(7453):1433–6.
2 Boynton PM, Greenhalgh T. A hands on guide to questionnaire research part one: selecting, designing, and developing your questionnaire. BMJ: British Medical Journal 2004;**328**(7451):1312–5.
3 Boynton PM. A hands on guide to questionnaire research part two: administering, analysing, and reporting your questionnaire. British Medical Journal 2004; **328**:1372–5.
4 Robson C. *Real world research: a resource for users of social research methods in applied settings.* Wiley: Chichester, 2011.
5 Bryman A. *Social research methods.* Oxford University Press, Oxford, 2012.
6 Dunn SM, Bryson JM, Hoskins PL, et al. Development of the diabetes knowledge (DKN) scales: forms DKNA, DKNB, and DKNC. Diabetes Care 1984;**7**(1):36–41.
7 Rahmqvist M, Bara A-C. Patient characteristics and quality dimensions related to patient satisfaction. International Journal for Quality in Health Care 2010; **22**(2):86–92.

8 Phillips D. *Quality of life: concept, policy and practice*. Routledge, London, 2012.
9 Bradley C, Speight J. Patient perceptions of diabetes and diabetes therapy: assessing quality of life. Diabetes/Metabolism Research and Reviews 2002;**18**(S3):S64–9.
10 Drewnowski A. Diet image: a new perspective on the food-frequency questionnaire. Nutrition Reviews 2001;**59**(11):370–2.
11 Adams AS, Soumerai SB, Lomas J, et al. Evidence of self-report bias in assessing adherence to guidelines. International Journal for Quality in Health Care 1999;**11**(3):187–92.
12 Gilbody S, House A, Sheldon T. Routine administration of Health Related Quality of Life (HRQoL) and needs assessment instruments to improve psychological outcome-a systematic review. Psychological Medicine 2002;**32**(8):1345–56.
13 Houtkoop-Steenstra H. *Interaction and the standardized survey interview: the living questionnaire*. Cambridge University Press, Cambridge, 2000.
14 Eysenbach G. Improving the quality of Web surveys: the Checklist for Reporting Results of Internet E-Surveys (CHERRIES). Journal of Medical Internet Research 2004;**6**(3):e34.
15 Draugalis JR, Coons SJ, Plaza CM. Best practices for survey research reports: a synopsis for authors and reviewers. American Journal of Pharmaceutical Education 2008;**72**(1):11.
16 Kelley K, Clark B, Brown V, et al. Good practice in the conduct and reporting of survey research. International Journal for Quality in Health Care 2003; **15**(3):261–6.
17 Bennett C, Khangura S, Brehaut JC, et al. Reporting guidelines for survey research: an analysis of published guidance and reporting practices. PLoS Medicine 2011;**8**(8):e1001069.

Chapter 14 **Papers that report quality improvement case studies**

What are quality improvement studies – and how should we research them?

The *British Medical Journal* (www.bmj.com) mainly publishes research articles. Another leading journal, *BMJ Quality and Safety* (http://qualitysafety .bmj.com), mainly publishes descriptions of efforts to improve the quality and safety of health care, often in real-world settings such as hospital wards or general practices [1]. If you are studying for an undergraduate exam, you should ask your tutors whether quality improvement studies are going to feature in your exams, because the material covered here is more often contained in postgraduate courses and you may find that it's not on your syllabus. If that is the case, put this chapter aside for after you've passed – you will certainly need it when you are working full time in the real world!

One key way of improving quality is to implement the findings of research and make care more evidence-based. This is discussed in the next chapter. But achieving a high-quality and safe health service requires more than evidence-based practice. Think of the last time you or one of your relatives was in hospital. I'm sure you wanted to have the most accurate diagnostic tests (Chapter 8), the most efficacious drugs (Chapter 6) or non-drug interventions (Chapter 7), and you also wanted the clinicians to follow evidence-based care plans and guidelines (Chapter 10) based on systematic reviews (Chapter 9). Furthermore, if the hospital asked you to help evaluate the service, you would have wanted them to use a valid and reliable questionnaire (Chapter 13).

But did you also care about things like how long you had to wait for an outpatient appointment and/or your operation, the attitudes of staff, the

How to Read a Paper: The Basics of Evidence-Based Medicine, Fifth Edition. Trisha Greenhalgh.
© 2014 John Wiley & Sons, Ltd. Published 2014 by John Wiley & Sons, Ltd.

clarity and completeness of the information you were given, the risk of catching an infection (e.g. when staff didn't wash their hands consistently), and the general efficiency of the place? If a member of staff made an error, was this openly disclosed to you and an unreserved apology offered? And if this happened, did the organisation have systems in place to learn from what went wrong and ensure it didn't happen again to someone else? A 'quality' health care experience includes all these things and more. The science of quality improvement draws its evidence from many different disciplines including research on manufacturing and air traffic control as well as evidence-based medicine [2–4].

Improving quality and safety in a particular area of health care typically involves a complex project lasting at least a few months, with input from different staff members (and increasingly, patients and their representatives, too) [5]. The leaders of the project help everyone involved set a goal and work towards it. The fortunes of the project are typically mixed – some things go well, other things not so well, and the initiative is typically written up (if at all) as a story.

For several years now, *BMJ* and *BMJ Quality & Safety* have distinguished research papers (presented as IMRAD – Introduction, Methods, Results and Discussion) from quality improvement reports (presented as COM-PASEN – Context, Outline of problem, Measures, Process, Analysis, Strategy for change, Effects of change, and Next steps). In making this distinction, research might be defined as *systematic and focused enquiry seeking truths that are transferable beyond the setting in which they were generated,* while quality improvement might be defined as *real-time, real-world work undertaken by teams who deliver services.*

You might have spotted that there is a large grey zone between these two activities. Some of this grey zone is quality improvement *research* – that is, applied research aimed at building the evidence base on how we should go about quality improvement studies. Quality improvement research embraces a broad range of methods including most of the ones described in the other chapters. In particular, the *mixed method case study* incorporates both quantitative data (e.g. measures of the prevalence of a particular condition or problem) and qualitative data (e.g. a careful analysis of the themes raised in complaint letters, or participant observation of staff going about their duties), all written up in an over-arching story about what was done, why, when, by whom and what the consequences were. If the paper is true quality improvement *research*, it should include a conclusion that offers transferable lessons for other teams in other settings [6, 7].

Incidentally, whilst the story ('anecdote') is rightly seen as a weak study design when, say, evaluating the efficacy of a drug, the story format ('organisational case study') has unique advantages when the task is to pull together a great deal of complex data and make sense of it, as is the case when an organisation sets out to improve its performance [8].

As you can probably imagine, critical appraisal of quality improvement research is a particularly challenging area. Unlike in randomised trials, there are not hard and fast rules on what the 'best' approach to a quality improvement initiative should be, and a great deal of subjective judgements may need to be made about the methods used and the significance of the findings. But as with all critical appraisal, the more papers you read and appraise, the better you will get.

In preparing the list of questions in the next section, I have drawn heavily on the SQUIRE (Standards for QUality Improvement Reporting Excellence) guidelines, which are the equivalent of Consolidated Standards of Reporting Trials (CONSORT), Preferred Reporting Items for Systematic Reviews and Meta-Analyses (PRISMA) and so on for quality improvement studies [9]. I was peripherally involved in the development of these guidelines, and I can confirm that they went through multiple iterations and struggles before appearing in print. This is because of the *inherent* challenges of producing structured checklists for appraising complex, multifaceted studies. To quote from the paper by the SQUIRE development group (p. 670):

> Unlike conceptually neat and procedurally unambiguous interventions, such as drugs, tests, and procedures, that directly affect the biology of disease and are the objects of study in most clinical research, improvement is essentially a social process. Improvement is an applied science rather than an academic discipline; its immediate purpose is to change human performance rather than generate new, generalizable knowledge, and it is driven primarily by experiential learning. Like other social processes, improvement is inherently context-dependent. [....] Although traditional experimental and quasiexperimental methods are important for learning <u>whether</u> improvement interventions change behavior, they do not provide appropriate and effective methods for addressing the crucial pragmatic ... questions [such as] What is it about the mechanism of a particular intervention that works, for whom does it work, and under what circumstances?

With these caveats in mind, let's see how far we can get with a checklist of questions to help make sense of quality improvement studies.

Ten questions to ask about a paper describing a quality improvement initiative

After I developed the following questions, I applied them to two recently published quality improvement studies, both of which I thought had some positive features but which might have scored even higher if the SQUIRE guidelines had been published when they were being written up. You might like to track down the papers and follow the examples. One is a study by Verdú et al. [10] from Spain, who wanted to improve the management of deep venous thrombosis (DVT) in hospital patients; and the other is a study by May et al. [11] from the USA, who sought to use academic detailing (which Wikipedia defines as 'non commercially based educational outreach', see section '"Evidence" and marketing') to improve evidence-based management of chronic illness in a primary care setting.

Question One: What was the context?

'Context' is the local detail of the real-world setting in which the work happened. Most obviously, one of our example studies happened in Spain, the other in the USA. One was in secondary care and the other in primary care. We will not be able to understand how these different initiatives unfolded without some background on the country, the health care system and (at a more local level) the particular historical, cultural, economic and micro-political aspects of our 'case'.

It is helpful, for example, not only to know that May et al.'s academic detailing study was targeted at private general practitioners (GPs) in the USA but also to read their brief description of the particular part of Kentucky where the doctors practised: 'This area has a regional metropolitan demography reflecting a considerable proportion of middle America (... population 260,512, median household income US $39,813, 19% non-White, 13% below the poverty line, one city, five rural communities and five historically black rural hamlets)' [11]. So this was an area – 'middle America' – which, overall, was neither especially affluent nor especially deprived, which included both urban and rural areas, and which was ethnically mixed but not dramatically so.

Question Two: What was the aim of the study?

It goes without saying that the aim of a quality improvement study is to improve quality! Perhaps the best way of framing this question is 'What was the problem for which the quality improvement initiative was seen as a solution?'

In Verdú et al.'s [10] DVT example, the authors are quite upfront that the aim of their quality improvement initiative was to save money!

More specifically, they sought to reduce the time patients spent in hospital ('length of stay'). In the academic detailing example, a 'rep' [UK terminology] or 'detailer' [US terminology] visited doctors to provide unbiased education and, in particular, to provide evidence-based guidelines for the management of diabetes (first visit) and chronic pain (second visit). The aim was to see whether the academic detailing model, which had been shown as long ago as 1983 to improve practice in *research* trials [11], could be made to work in the messier and less predictable environment of real-world middle America.

Question Three: What was the mechanism by which the authors hoped to improve quality?

This HOW question is all-important. Look back to section 'Ten questions to ask about a paper describing a complex intervention' on complex interventions, when I asked (Question Four) 'What was the theoretical mechanism of action of the intervention?'. This is effectively the same question, although quality improvement initiatives typically have fuzzy boundaries and you should not necessarily expect to identify a clear 'core' to the intervention.

In the DVT care pathway example, the logic behind the initiative was that if they developed an integrated care pathway incorporating all the relevant evidence-based tests and treatments in the right order, stipulating who was responsible for each step, and excluding anything for which there was evidence of no benefit, staff would follow it. In consequence, the patient would spend less time in hospital and have fewer unnecessary procedures. Furthermore, sharpening up the pathway would, they hoped, also reduce adverse events (such as haemorrhage).

In the academic detailing example, the 'mechanism' for changing doctors' prescribing behaviour was the principles of interpersonal influence and persuasion on which the pharmaceutical industry has built its marketing strategy (and which I spent much of Chapter 6 warning you about). Personally supplying the guidelines and talking the doctors through them would, it was hoped, increase the chance that they would be followed.

Question Four: Was the intended quality improvement initiative evidence-based?

Some measures aimed at improving quality seem like a good idea in theory but actually don't work in practice. Perhaps the best example of this is mergers – that is, joining two small health care organisations (e.g. hospitals) with the aim of achieving efficiency savings, economies of scale, and so on. Fulop's [12] team demonstrated that not only do such savings rarely materialise but merged organisations often encounter new, unanticipated problems. In this example, there is not merely no evidence of benefit but evidence that the initiative might cause harm!

In the DVT example, there is a systematic review demonstrating that overall, in the research setting, developing and implementing integrated care pathways (also known as *critical care pathways*) *can* reduce costs and length of stay [13]. Similarly, systematic reviews have confirmed the efficacy of academic detailing in research trials [14]. In both of our examples, then, the '*can* it work?' question had been answered and the authors were asking a more specific and contextualised question: '*does* it work here, with *these* people and *this* particular set of constraints and contingencies?' [15].

Question Five: How did the authors measure success, and was this reasonable?

At a recent conference, I wandered around a poster exhibition in which groups of evidence-based medicine enthusiasts were presenting their attempts to improve the quality of a service. I was impressed by some, but very disheartened to find that not uncommonly the authors had not formally measured the success of their initiative at all – or even defined what 'success' would look like!

Our two case examples did better. Verdú et al. evaluated their DVT study in terms of six outcomes: length of hospital stay, cost of the hospital care, and what they called as *care indicators* (the proportion of patients whose care actually followed the pathway; the proportion whose length of stay was actually reduced in line with the pathway's recommendations; the rate of adverse events; and the level of patient satisfaction). Taken together, these gave a fair indication of whether the quality improvement initiative was a success. However, it was not perfect – for example, the satisfaction questionnaire would not have shaped up well against the criteria for a good questionnaire study in Chapter 13.

In the academic detailing example, a good measure of the success of the initiative would surely have been the extent to which the doctors followed the guidelines or (even better) the impact on patients' health and well-being. But these downstream, patient-relevant outcome measures were not used. Instead, the authors' definition of 'success' was much more modest: they simply wanted their evidence-based detailers to get a regular foot in the door of the private GPs. To that end, their outcome measures included the proportion of doctors in the area who agreed to be visited at all; the duration of the visit (being shown the door after 45 s would be a 'failed' visit); whether the doctor agreed to be seen on a second or subsequent occasion; and if so, whether he or she could readily locate the guidelines supplied at the first visit.

It could be argued that these measures are the equivalent of the 'surrogate endpoints' I discussed in section 'surrogate endpoints'. But given the real-world context (a target group of geographically and professionally isolated private practitioners steeped in pharmaceutical industry advertising, for whom evidence-based practice was not traditionally part of their core business), a 'foot in the door' is a lot better than nothing. Nevertheless, when appraising the paper, we should be clear about the authors' modest definition of success and interpret the conclusions accordingly.

Question Six: How much detail was given about the change process, and what insights can be gleaned from this?

The devil of a change effort is often in the nitty-gritty detail. In the DVT care pathway example, the methods section was fairly short and left me hungry for more. Although I liked many aspects of the paper, I was irritated by this briefest of descriptions of what was actually done to *develop* the pathway: 'After the design of the clinical pathway, we started the study . . . .'. But *who* designed the pathway, and how? Experts in evidence-based practice – or people working at the front line of care? Ideally, it would have been both, but we don't know. Were just the doctors involved – or were nurses, pharmacists, patients and others (such as or the hospital's director of finance) included in the process? Were there arguments about the evidence – or did everyone agree on what was needed? The more information about *process* we can find in the paper, the more we can interpret both positive and negative findings.

In the academic detailing example, the methods section is very long and includes details on how the programme of 'detailing' was developed, how the detailers were selected and trained, how the sample of doctors was chosen, how the detailers approached the doctors, what supporting materials were used, and how the detailing visits were structured and adapted to the needs and learning styles of different doctors. Whether we agree with their measures of the project's success or not, we can certainly interpret the findings in the light of this detailed information on how they went about it.

The relatively short methods section in the DVT care pathway example may have been a victim of the word length requirements of the journal. Authors summarise their methods in order to appear succinct, and thereby leave out all the qualitative detail that would allow you to evaluate the *process* of quality improvement – that is, to build up a 'rich picture' of what the authors actually did. In recognition of this perverse incentive, the authors of the SQUIRE guidelines issued a plea to editors for 'longer papers' [9]. A well-written quality improvement study might run into a dozen or more pages, and it will generally take you a lot longer to read than, say, a tightly written report on a randomised trial. The increasing tendency for journals to include 'eXtra' (with the 'e' meaning 'online') material in an Internet-accessible format is extremely encouraging, and you should hunt such material down whenever it is available.

Question Seven: What were the main findings?

For this question you need to return to your answer to Question Five and find the numbers (for quantitative outcomes) or the key themes (for qualitative data), and ask whether and how these were significant. Just as in other study designs, 'significance' in quality improvement case studies is a multifaceted concept. A change in a numerical value may be clinically significant without being statistically significant or vice versa (see section 'Probability and confidence'), and may also be vulnerable to various biases. For example, in a before and after study, time will have moved on between the 'baseline' and 'post intervention' measures, and a host of confounding variables including the economic climate, public attitudes, availability of particular drugs or procedures, relevant case law, and the identity of the chief executive, may have changed. Qualitative outcomes may be particularly vulnerable to the Hawthorne effect (staff tend to feel valued and work harder when any change in working conditions aimed at improving performance is introduced, whether it has any intrinsic merits or not) [16].

In the DVT care pathway example, mean length of stay was reduced by 2 days (a difference that was statistically significant), and financial savings were achieved of several hundred Euros per patient. Furthermore, 40 of 42 eligible patients were actually cared for using the new care pathway (a further 18 patients with DVT did not meet the inclusion criteria), and 62% of all patients achieved the target reduction in length of stay. Overall, 7 of 60 people experienced adverse events, and in only one of these had the care pathway been followed. These figures, taken together, not only tell us that the initiative achieved the goal of saving money but they also give us a clear indication of the extent to which the intended changes in the process of care were achieved *and* remind us that many patients with DVT are what are known as *exceptions* – that is, management by a standardised pathway doesn't suit their needs.

In the academic detailing example, the findings show that of the 130 doctors in the target group, 78% received at least one visit and these people did not differ in demographic characteristics (e.g. age, sex, whether qualified abroad or not) from those who refused a visit. Only one person refused point blank to receive further visits, but getting another visit scheduled proved challenging, and barriers were 'primarily associated with persuading office staff of the physician's stated intentions for further visits'. In other words, even though the doctor was (allegedly) keen, the detailers had trouble getting past the receptionists – surely a significant qualitative finding about the process of academic detailing, which had not been uncovered in the randomised trial design! Half the doctors could lay their hands on the guidelines at the second visit (and by implication, half couldn't). But the paper also presented some questionable quantitative outcome data such as 'around 90% of practitioners appeared interested in the topics discussed' – an observation which, apart from being entirely subjective, is a Hawthorne effect until proved otherwise. Rather than using the dubious technique of trying to quantify their subjective impressions, perhaps the authors should have either stuck to their primary outcome measure (whether the doctors let them in the door or not) or gone the whole hog and measured compliance with the guidelines.

Question Eight: What was the explanation for the success, failure or mixed fortunes of the initiative – and was this reasonable?

Once again, conventions on the length of papers in journals may make this section frustratingly short. Ideally, the authors will have considered their findings, revisited the contextual factors you identified in Question One, and offered a plausible and reasoned explanation for the former in terms of the latter, including a consideration of alternative explanations. More commonly, explanations are brief and speculative.

Why, for example, was it difficult for academic detailers to gain access to doctors for second appointments? According to the authors, the difficulty was because of 'customarily short open-diary times for future appointments and operational factors related to the lack of permanent funding for this service'. But an alternative explanation might have been that the doctor was disinterested but did not wish to be confrontational, so told the receptionists to stall if approached again!

As in this example, evaluating the explanations given in a paper for disappointing outcomes in a quality improvement project is always a judgement call. Nobody is going to be able to give you a checklist that will allow you to say with 100% accuracy '*this* explanation was definitely plausible, whereas *that* aspect definitely wasn't'. In a quality improvement case study, the authors of the paper will have told a story about what happened, and you will have to interpret their story using your knowledge of evidence-based medicine, your knowledge of people and organisations, and your common sense.

The DVT care pathway paper, whilst offering very positive findings, offers a realistic explanation of them: 'The real impact of clinical pathways on length of stay is difficult to ascertain because these non-randomised, partly retrospective, studies might show significant reductions in hospital stay but cannot prove that the only cause of the reduction is the clinical pathway'. Absolutely!

Question Nine: In the light of the findings, what do the authors feel are the next steps in the quality improvement cycle locally?

Quality is not a station you arrive at but a manner of travelling. (If you want a reference for that statement, the best I can offer is Pirsig's [17] 'Zen and the Art of Motorcycle Maintenance'). To put it another way, quality improvement is a never-ending cycle: when you reach one goal, you set yourself another.

The DVT care pathway team were pleased that they had significantly reduced length of stay, and felt that the way to improve further was to ensure that the care pathway was modified promptly as new evidence and new technologies became available. Another approach, which they did not mention but which would not need to wait for an innovation, might be to apply the care pathway approach to a different medical or surgical condition.

The academic detailing team decided that their next step would be to change the curriculum slightly so that rather than covering two unrelated topics on different topic areas, they would use 'judicious selection of sequential topics allowing subtle reflection of key message elements from previous encounters (e.g. management of diabetes followed by a programme on management of hypertension)'. It is interesting that they did not consider addressing the problem of attrition (42% of doctors did not make themselves available for the second visit).

Question Ten: What did the authors claim to be the generalisable lessons for other teams, and was this reasonable?

At the beginning of this chapter, I argued that the hallmark of research was generalisable lessons for others. There is nothing wrong with improving quality locally without seeking to generate wider lessons, but if the authors have published their work, they are often claiming that others should follow their approach – or at least, selected aspects of it.

In the DVT care pathway example, the authors make no claims about the transferability of their findings. Their sample size was small, and care pathways have already been shown to shorten hospital stay in other comparable conditions. Their reason for publishing appears to convey the message, 'If we could do it, so can you'!

In the academic detailing example, the potentially transferable finding was said to be that a whole population approach to academic detailing (i.e. seeking access to every GP in a particular geographical area) as opposed to only targeting volunteers, can 'work'. This claim could be true, but because the outcome measures were subjective and not directly relevant to patients, this study fell short of demonstrating it.

Conclusion

In this chapter, I have tried to guide you through how to make judgements about papers on quality improvement studies. As the quote at the end of section 'What are quality improvement studies – and how should we research them?' illustrates, such judgements are inherently difficult to make and require you to integrate evidence and information from multiple sources. Hence, whilst quality improvement studies are often small, local and even somewhat parochial, critically appraising such studies is often more of a headache than appraising a large meta-analysis!

References

1 Batalden PB, Davidoff F. What is "quality improvement" and how can it transform healthcare? Quality and Safety in Health Care 2007;**16**(1):2–3.

2 Marshall M. Applying quality improvement approaches to health care. BMJ: British Medical Journal 2009;339:b3411.

3 Miltner RS, Newsom JH, Mittman BS. The future of quality improvement research. Implementation Science 2013;**8**(Suppl 1):S9.

4 Vincent C, Batalden P, Davidoff F. Multidisciplinary centres for safety and quality improvement: learning from climate change science. BMJ Quality & Safety 2011;**20**(Suppl 1):i73–8.

5 Alexander JA, Hearld LR. The science of quality improvement implementation: developing capacity to make a difference. Medical Care 2011;**49**:S6–20.

6 Casarett D, Karlawish JH, Sugarman J. Determining when quality improvement initiatives should be considered research. JAMA: The Journal of the American Medical Association 2000;**283**(17):2275–80.

7 Lynn J. When does quality improvement count as research? Human subject protection and theories of knowledge. Quality and Safety in Health Care 2004; **13**(1):67–70.

8 Greenhalgh T, Russell J, Swinglehurst D. Narrative methods in quality improvement research. Quality & Safety in Health Care 2005;**14**(6):443–9 doi: 10.1136/qshc.2005.014712[published Online First: Epub Date].

9 Davidoff F, Batalden P, Stevens D, et al. Publication guidelines for improvement studies in health care: evolution of the SQUIRE Project. Annals of Internal Medicine 2008;**149**(9):670–6.

10 Verdú A, Maestre A, López P, et al. Clinical pathways as a healthcare tool: design, implementation and assessment of a clinical pathway for lower-extremity deep venous thrombosis. Quality and Safety in Health Care 2009;**18**(4):314–20.

11　May F, Simpson D, Hart L, et al. Experience with academic detailing services for quality improvement in primary care practice. Quality and Safety in Health Care 2009;**18**(3):225–31.

12　Fulop N, Protopsaltis G, King A, et al. Changing organisations: a study of the context and processes of mergers of health care providers in England. Social Science & Medicine 2005;**60**(1):119–30.

13　Rotter T, Kinsman L, James E, et al. Clinical pathways: effects on professional practice, patient outcomes, length of stay and hospital costs. Cochrane Database of Systematic Reviews (Online) 2010;**3**(3) doi: 10.1002/14651858.CD006632.pub2.

14　O'Brien M, Rogers S, Jamtvedt G, et al. Educational outreach visits: effects on professional practice and health care outcomes. Cochrane Database of Systematic Reviews (Online) 2007;**4**(4):1–62.

15　Haynes B. Can it work? Does it work? Is it worth it?: the testing of healthcare interventions is evolving. BMJ: British Medical Journal 1999;**319**(7211):652–63.

16　Franke RH, Kaul JD. The Hawthorne experiments: first statistical interpretation. American Sociological Review 1978:623–43.

17　Pirsig R. *Zen and the art of motorcycle maintenance: an enquiry into values.* New York: Bantam Books, 1984.

Chapter 15 **Getting evidence into practice**

Why are health professionals slow to adopt evidence-based practice?

Health professionals' failure to practice in accordance with the best available evidence cannot be attributed entirely to ignorance or stubbornness. Consultant paediatrician Dr Van Someren [1] has described a (now historical) example that illustrates many of the additional barriers to getting research evidence into practice: the prevention of neonatal respiratory distress syndrome in premature babies.

It was discovered back in 1957 that babies born more than 6 weeks early may get into severe breathing difficulties because of lack of a substance called *surfactant*, which lowers the surface tension within the lung alveoli and reduces resistance to expansion. Pharmaceutical companies began research in the 1960s to develop an artificial surfactant that could be given to the infant to prevent the life-threatening syndrome developing, but it was not until the mid-1980s that an effective product was developed.

By the late 1980s, a number of randomised trials had taken place, and a meta-analysis published in 1990 suggested that the benefits of artificial surfactant greatly outweighed its risks. In 1990, a 6000-patient trial (OSIRIS) was begun, involving almost all the major neonatal intensive care units in the UK. The manufacturer was awarded a product licence in 1990, and by 1993, practically every eligible premature infant in the UK was receiving artificial surfactant.

Another treatment had also been shown a generation previously to prevent neonatal respiratory distress syndrome: administration of the steroid drug dexamethasone to mothers in premature labour. Dexamethasone worked by accelerating the rate at which the foetal lung reached maturity. Its efficacy had been demonstrated in experimental animals in 1969, and in clinical trials on

---

How to Read a Paper: The Basics of Evidence-Based Medicine, Fifth Edition. Trisha Greenhalgh.
© 2014 John Wiley & Sons, Ltd. Published 2014 by John Wiley & Sons, Ltd.

humans, published in the prestigious journal *Paediatrics*, as early as 1972. Yet, despite a significant beneficial effect being confirmed in a number of further trials, and a meta-analysis published in 1990, the take-up of this technology was astonishingly slow. It was estimated in 1995 that only 12–18% of eligible mothers were receiving this treatment in the USA [2].

The quality of the evidence and the magnitude of the effect were similar for both these interventions [3, 4]. Why were the paediatricians so much quicker than the obstetricians at implementing an intervention that prevented avoidable deaths? Dr Van Someren [1] considered a number of factors, listed in Table 15.1. The effect of artificial surfactant is virtually immediate, and the doctor administering it witnesses directly the 'cure' of a terminally sick baby. Pharmaceutical industry support for a large (and, arguably, scientifically unnecessary) trial ensured that few consultant paediatricians appointed in the early 1990s would have escaped being introduced to the new technology.

In contrast, steroids, particularly for pregnant women, were unfashionable and perceived by patients to be 'bad for you'. In doctors' eyes, dexamethasone was an old hat treatment for a host of unglamorous diseases, notably end-stage cancer, and the scientific mechanism for its effect on foetal lungs was not readily understood. Most poignantly of all, an obstetrician would rarely get a chance to witness directly the life-saving effect on an individual patient.

Table 15.1 Factors influencing implementation of evidence to prevent neonatal respiratory distress syndrome (Dr V Van Someren, personal communication)

	Surfactant treatment	Prenatal steroid treatment
Perception of mechanism	Corrects a surfactant deficiency disease	Ill-defined effect on developing lung tissue
Timing of effect	Minutes	Days
Impact on prescriber	Views effect directly (has to stand by ventilator)	Sees effect as statistic in annual report
Perception of side effects	Perceived as minimal	Clinicians' and patients' anxiety disproportionate to actual risk
Conflict between two patients	No (paediatrician's patient will benefit directly)	Yes (obstetrician's patient will not benefit directly)
Pharmaceutical industry interest	High (patented product; huge potential revenue)	Low (product out of patent; small potential revenue)
Trial technology	'New' (developed in late 1980s)	'Old' (developed in early 1970s)
Widespread involvement of clinicians in trials	Yes	No

The above-mentioned example is far from isolated. Effective health care strategies frequently (although, thankfully, not always) take years to catch on, even amongst the experts who should be at the cutting edge of practice [5–8]. The remaining sections in this chapter consider how we can reduce the time from research evidence appearing to making real differences in health outcomes. Be warned – there are no quick fixes.

How much avoidable suffering is caused by failing to implement evidence?

The short answer to this question is 'a lot'. I recently discovered a paper by Woolf and Johnson [9] in the *Annals of Family Medicine*, entitled: 'The break-even point: when medical advances are less important than improving the fidelity with which they are delivered'. Their argument is this. Imagine a disease that kills 100 000 people a year. If we demonstrate through research that drug X is effective for this disease, reducing mortality by 20%, it will potentially save 20 000 lives per year. But if only 50% of eligible patients actually receive the drug, the number of lives saved is reduced to 10 000. They argue that in many cases, we would add more value by increasing our efforts to implement this evidence than by doing more research to develop a different drug whose efficacy is greater than drug X.

If you think these figures are speculative, here's a real example quoted from Woolf and Johnson's paper, in which they cite evidence from a meta-analysis of the impact of aspirin in acute stroke and a survey of prescribing practice in the USA:

> *A systematic review by the Antithrombotic Trialists Collaboration reported that the use of aspirin by patients who had previously experienced a stroke or transient ischemic attack reduces the incidence of recurrent nonfatal strokes by 23%. That is, in a population in which 100,000 people were destined to have strokes, 23,000 events could be prevented if all eligible patients took aspirin. McGlynn et al.1 reported, however, that antiplatelet therapy is given to only 58% of eligible patients. At that rate, only 13,340 strokes would be prevented in the hypothetical population, whereas achieving 100% fidelity in offering aspirin would prevent 23,000 strokes (i.e., 9,660 additional strokes) [9].*

In summary, the amount of avoidable suffering caused by failure to implement evidence is unknown – but it could be calculated using the method set out in Woolf and Johnson's paper. It is encouraging that a growing (although still small) proportion of research funding is now allocated to increasing the proportion of patients who benefit from things we know work.

How can we influence health professionals' behaviour to promote evidence-based practice?

The Cochrane Effective Practice and Organisation of Care Group (EPOC, described in Chapter 10 and online at http://epoc.cochrane.org) have done a thorough job of summarising the literature accumulated from research trials on what is and is not effective in changing professional practice – both in promoting effective innovations and in encouraging professionals to resist 'innovations' that are ineffective or harmful. EPOC have been mainly interested in reviewing trials of interventions aimed at redressing potential gaps in the evidence-into-practice sequence.

One of the few unequivocal messages from EPOC's work is that simply *telling* people about evidence-based medicine (EBM) is consistently ineffective at changing practice. Until relatively recently, education (at least in relation to the training of doctors) was more or less synonymous with the didactic talk-and-chalk sessions that most of us remember from school and college. The 'bums on seats' approach to postgraduate education (filling lecture theatres up with doctors or nurses and wheeling on an 'expert' to impart pearls of wisdom) is relatively cheap and convenient for the educators but does not generally lead to sustained behaviour change in practice. Indeed, one study demonstrated that the number of reported 'CME' (continuing medical education) hours attended was *inversely* correlated with doctors' competence [10]!

If, like me, you are interested in the theory underpinning EBM teaching, you will have spotted that the 'instructional' approach to promoting professional behaviour change in relation to EBM is built on the flawed assumption that people behave in a particular way *because (and only because) they lack knowledge*, and that imparting knowledge will therefore change behaviour. Marteau and colleagues' [10] short and authoritative critique shows that this model has neither theoretical coherence nor empirical support. Information, they conclude, may be *necessary* for professional behaviour change, but it is rarely, if ever, *sufficient*. Given here are psychological theories that Marteau and her team felt might inform the design of more effective educational strategies.

- *Behavioural learning*: The notion that behaviour is more likely to be repeated if it is associated with rewards, and less likely if it is punished.
- *Social cognition*: When planning an action, individuals ask themselves 'Is it worth the cost?', 'What do other people think about this?' and 'Am I capable of achieving it?'.
- *Stages of change models*: In these, all individuals are considered to lie somewhere on a continuum of readiness to change from no awareness that there is a need to change through to sustained implementation of the desired behaviour.

More recently, Michie's [11] team extended this simple taxonomy with a smorgasbord of other behaviour change theories taken from cognitive psychology, and Eccles's [12] team (which includes guideline guru Jeremy Grimshaw) applied a similar set of psychological theories specifically to uptake of evidence-based practice by doctors.

What sort of educational approaches have actually been shown to be effective for promoting evidence-based practice? Here's a summary of the empirical literature, based mainly on four systematic reviews of intervention trials [13–16].

(a) EBM teaching as conventionally delivered in undergraduate medical education curricula improves students' EBM knowledge and attitudes, but an impact on their performance in dealing with real cases has not been convincingly demonstrated.

(b) In relation to qualified doctors, most classroom-based EBM training has little or no impact on their knowledge or critical appraisal skills. This may be because both the training and the tests are non-compulsory; or it may be because the training itself is too little, too superficial, too formulaic, too passive and too removed from practice.

(c) More educationally sound approaches such as 'integrated' EBM teaching (e.g. during ward rounds or in the emergency room) or intensive short courses using highly interactive learning methods can produce significant changes in knowledge, skills and behaviour.

(d) However, no direct impact has yet been demonstrated from such courses on any patient-relevant outcomes.

Green [17, 18], who has conducted one of the most rigorous primary studies of EBM training ever organised, as well as a national survey of programmes and a critical overview, holds the view that EBM teaching should occur 'where the rubber meets the road' – that is, in the clinic and at the bedside . He cites adult learning theory to support the argument that EBM teaching must surely be more effective if the learner can relate it to practical problems in the here-and-now and use it for real (as opposed to hypothetical) decision making – and he has also undertaken qualitative work to confirm that these real-world practical barriers (lack of time, evidence inaccessible when it is needed, unforgiving organisational culture, etc.) account for much of the theory–practice gap in EBM implementation [19]. The way forward, he suggests, is for more work to be carried out ensuring that evidence is available and readily accessible at the point of care, enabling clinical questions to be raised and answered in a context that optimises active learning.

In Chapter 10, I described the main findings of Grimshaw's [20] 2004 systematic review on guideline implementation. The main conclusion of that review was that despite hundreds of studies costing millions of dollars, no intervention, either educational or otherwise, and either singly or in combination, is *guaranteed* to change the behaviour of practitioners in an 'evidence-based' direction.

Here's where I part company slightly with the EPOC approach. While many EPOC members are still undertaking trials (and reviews of trials) to add to the research base on whether this or that intervention (such leaflets and other printed educational materials [21], audit and feedback [22] or financial incentives [23, 24]) is or is not effective in changing clinician behaviour, my own view is that this endeavour is misplaced. Not only have no magic bullets been identified yet, but I believe *they never will be identified* – and that we should stop looking for them.

This is because the implementation of best practice is highly complex; it involves multiple influences operating in different directions [25]; and it is dependent on *people*. An approach that has a positive effect in one study might have a negative effect in another study, so the notion of an 'effect size' of an intervention to change clinician behaviour is not only meaningless but actively misleading. If you have children, you'll know that a childrearing strategy that worked well for your first child might not have worked at all for your second child, for reasons you can't easily explain. It's something to do with human quirkiness (child two is a different individual with a different personality), and also to do with the fact that the context is subtly different in multiple ways, even in the 'same' family environment (child two has an older sibling, busier parents, hand-me-down toys, etc.). So it is with organisations, their staff, and evidence-based practice. Even the more refined research approach of looking for 'mediators' and 'moderators' of the effectiveness of particular interventions [12] is still, in my view, based on the flawed assumption that there is a consistent 'mediator/moderator effect' from a particular contextual variable.

Let's think a bit more about the human factor. In a systematic review of the diffusion of organisational-level innovations in health services, I drew this conclusion about the human elements in the adoption of innovations.

People are not passive recipients of innovations. Rather (and to a greater or lesser extent in different individuals), they seek innovations out, experiment with them, evaluate them, find (or fail to find) meaning in them, develop feelings (positive or negative) about them, challenge them, worry about them, complain about them, 'work round' them, talk to others about them, develop know-how about them, modify them to fit particular tasks, and attempt to improve or redesign them [25].

These were the key factors my team found to be associated with a person's readiness to adopt health care innovations.

(a) *General psychological antecedents*: A number of personality traits are associated with the propensity to try out and use innovations (e.g. tolerance of ambiguity, intellectual ability, motivation, values and learning style). In short, some people are more set in their ways than others – and these individuals will need more input and take more time to change.

(b) *Context-specific psychological antecedents*: A person who is motivated and capable (in terms of values, goals, specific skills, etc.) to use a particular innovation is more likely to adopt it. Also, if the innovation meets an *identified need* in the intended adopter, they are more likely to adopt it.

(c) *Meaning*: The meaning that the innovation holds for the person has a powerful influence on his or her decision to adopt it. The meaning attached to an innovation is generally not fixed but can be negotiated and reframed – for example, through discussions with other professionals or others within the organisation. For example, in the example described in section 'The rise and rise of questionnaire research', one of the problems was probably that dexamethasone therapy was unconsciously seen by doctors as 'an old-fashioned palliative care drug, used in older people'. In changing their practice, they had to place this therapy in a new mental schema – as 'an up-to-date preventive therapy, appropriate for pregnant women'.

(d) *Nature of the adoption decision*: The decision by an individual in an organisation to adopt a particular innovation is rarely independent of other decisions. It may be contingent (dependent on a decision made by someone else in the organisation); collective (the individual has a 'vote' but ultimately must follow the decision of a group); or authoritative (the individual is told whether to adopt or not). A good example of promoting evidence-based practice through an authoritative adoption decision is the development of hospital or practice formularies. Drugs of marginal value or poor cost-effectiveness ratio can be removed from the list of drugs that the hospital is prepared to pay for. But (as you may have discovered if you work with an imposed formulary), such policies also inhibit evidence-based practice because the innovator who is ahead of the game must wait (sometimes years) for a committee decision before implementing a new standard of practice.

(e) *Concerns and information needs*: People are concerned about different things at different stages in the adoption of an innovation. Initially, they need *general information* (what is the new 'evidence-based' practice, what does it cost, and how might it affect me?); in the early adoption stages, they need *hands-on information* (how do I make it work in practice?), and as they become more confident in the new practice, they need *development and adaptation information* (can I adapt this practice a bit to suit my circumstances, and if so, how should I do that?).

Having explored the nature of human idiosyncracy, another important factor to consider is the influence one person can have on another. As Rogers [26] first demonstrated in relation to the adoption of agricultural innovations by Iowa farmers (who are perhaps even more set in their ways than doctors), interpersonal contact is the most powerful method of influence. The main type of interpersonal influence relevant to the adoption of evidence-based practice is the *opinion leader*. We copy two sorts of people: people we look up to ('expert opinion leaders') and people we think are just like us ('peer opinion leaders') [27].

An opinion leader who is opposed to a new practice – or even one who is lukewarm and fails to back it – has a great deal of potential wrecking power. But as this systematic review of opinion leader intervention trials showed, just because a doctor is more likely to change his or her prescribing behaviour if a respected opinion leader has already changed, it doesn't necessarily follow that targeting opinion leaders (doctors nominated by other doctors as individuals they would consult or copy) with educational interventions will lead to a widespread change in prescribing practice [28]. This is probably because opinion leaders have minds of their own, and also because of the many other influences on practice apart from that one individual. In the real world, so-called 'social influence policies' may fail to influence.

Another important model of interpersonal influence, which the pharmaceutical industry has shown to be highly effective, is one-to-one contact between doctors and drug company representatives (discussed in Chapter 6 and known in the UK as 'reps' and the USA as 'detailers'), whose influence on clinical behaviour may be so dramatic that they have been dubbed the 'stealth bombers' of medicine. As the example in section 'Ten questions to ask about a paper describing a quality improvement initiative' shows, this tactic has been harnessed by non-commercial change agencies in what is known as *academic detailing*: the educator books in to see the physician in the same way as industry representatives, but in this case the 'rep' provides objective, complete and comparative information about a range of different drugs and encourages the clinician to adopt a critical approach to the evidence. Whilst dramatic short-term changes in practice have been demonstrated in research trials, the example in the previous chapter shows that in a real-world setting, consistent [29], positive changes to patient care may be hard to demonstrate. As ever, the intervention should not be seen as a panacea.

A final approach to note in relation to supporting implementation of evidence-based practice is the use of computerised decision support systems that incorporate the research evidence and can be accessed by the busy practitioner at the touch of a button. Dozens of these systems are currently being developed, piloted and tested in randomised controlled trials. Relatively few are in routine use. There have been several systematic reviews of such systems, for example, Garg et al.'s [30] synthesis of 100 empirical studies published in *JAMA*, and Black et al.'s [31] 'review of reviews' covering 13 previous systematic reviews on clinical decision support. Garg et al. showed that around two-thirds of these studies demonstrated improved clinical performance in the decision support arm, with the best results being in drug dosing and active clinical care (e.g. management of asthma) and the worst results in diagnosis. Systems that included a spontaneous prompt (as opposed to requiring the clinician to activate the system) and those in which the trial was conducted by the people who developed the technology (as opposed to using an 'off-the-shelf' product) were the most effective. Black et al.'s more recent review broadly confirmed these findings. Most, but not studies, seemed to show significant improvements in clinical performance (e.g. following a guideline, actioning preventive care such as immunisation or cancer screening) with computerised decision support, but the impact on patient outcomes was much more variable. The latter were only measured in around a quarter of studies, and where they were, they usually showed modest or absent impact except in post-hoc subgroup analyses (which have questionable statistical validity).

Note what I said earlier (page 207) about the complexity of the implementation of EBM. I am sceptical of studies that attempt to say 'computer-based decision support is/is not effective' or 'computer-based decision support has an effect of X magnitude'. They work for some people in some circumstances, and our research energies should now be directed at refining what we can say about *what sort of* computerised decision support, *for whom* and *in what circumstances* [32]. Resistance to new technologies by clinicians is one of my current research interests – but if I told you the whole story here I would never finish this book, so if you are interested, make a note to look out some of my in-progress work in a year or so.

What does an 'evidence-based organisation' look like?

'What does an organisation that promotes the adoption of [evidence-based] innovations look like?' was one of the questions that my own team addressed in our systematic review of the literature on diffusion of organisational-level innovations [25]. We found that, in general, an organisation will assimilate a new product or practice more readily if it is large, mature (has been established a long time), functionally differentiated (i.e. divided into semi-autonomous departments and units), specialised (a well-developed division of labour, such as specialist services); if it has slack resources (money and staff) to channel into new projects; and if it has decentralised decision-making structures (teams can work autonomously). But although dozens of studies (and five meta-analyses) have been undertaken on the size and structure of organisations, all these determinants account for less than 15% of the variation in organisations' ability to support innovation (and in many studies, they explain none of the variation at all). In other words, it's not usually the structure of the organisation that makes the critical difference in supporting EBM.

More important in our review were less easily measurable dimensions of the organisation – particularly something the organisational theorists call *absorptive capacity*. Absorptive capacity is defined as the organisation's ability to identify, capture, interpret, share, reframe and re-codify new knowledge, to link it with its own existing knowledge base, and to put it to appropriate use [33]. Prerequisites for absorptive capacity include the organisation's existing knowledge and skills base (especially its store of tacit, 'knowing the ropes' type knowledge) and pre-existing related technologies; a 'learning organisation' culture (in which people are encouraged to learn amongst themselves and share knowledge); and proactive leadership directed towards enabling this knowledge sharing [34].

A major overview by Dopson and her colleagues [35] of high-quality quali- tative studies on how research evidence is identified, circulated, evaluated and used in health care organisations found that that before it can be fully imple- mented in an organisation, EBM knowledge must be enacted and made social, entering into the stock of knowledge that is developed and socially shared amongst others in the organisation. In other words, knowledge depends for its circulation on interpersonal networks (who knows whom), and will only spread efficiently through the organisation if these social features are taken into account and barriers overcome.

Another difficult-to-measure dimension of the evidence-based organisa- tion (i.e. one that is capable of capturing best practice and implementing it widely in the organisation) is what is known and a *receptive context for change*. This composite construct, developed in relation to the implementation of best practice in healthcare by Pettigrew and colleagues [36], incorporates a num- ber of organisational features that have been independently associated with its ability to embrace new ideas and face the prospect of change. In addition to absorptive capacity for new knowledge (see preceding text), the compo- nents of receptive context include strong leadership, clear strategic vision, good managerial relations, visionary staff in key positions, a climate con- ducive to experimentation and risk-taking, and effective data capture systems.

Leadership may be especially critical in encouraging organisational members to break out of the convergent thinking and routines that are the norm in large, well-established organisations.

Another paper that's worth looking up is Gustafson's [37] quasi-systematic review of the determinants of successful change projects in health care organisations. The 18 items in Gustafson's final model include:

- tension for change (staff feel that current practice is sub-optimal and want things to be different);
- balance of power (staff supporting the change outnumber, and are more strategically placed in the organisation, than staff opposing it);
- perceived advantages (everyone understands the change and believes its advantages outweigh the disadvantages);
- flexibility (the new practice can be adapted to fit local needs and ways of working);
- time and resources (the change is adequately funded and people have protected time to work on it).

If this sounds like a recipe your organisation can't follow in relation to EBM, read the next section (and if that doesn't help, consider changing jobs!).

For those with an appetite for 'hard core' management and organisation studies papers, I recommend Ferlie's [38] team's recent summary of the literature on such topics as knowledge as a resource in organisations (known in the jargon as the 'resource-based view of the firm') and critical management studies (a field of research that asks questions such as 'who holds the power in this organisation?' and 'whose interests does this change serve?'), applied to the question of whether and how quickly organisations adopt evidence-based practices and policies. Their findings are diverse, hence difficult to summarise, but it is clear that the EBM community has much to learn from our colleagues in management disciplines.

How can we help organisations develop the appropriate structures, systems and values to support evidence-based practice?

Whilst there is a wealth of evidence on the sort of organisation that supports evidence-based practice, there is much less evidence on the effectiveness of specific interventions to *change* an organisation to make it more 'evidence based' – and it is beyond the scope of this book to address this topic comprehensively. Much of the literature on organisational change is in the form of practical checklists or the 'ten tips for success' type format. Checklists and tips can be enormously useful, but such lists tend to leave me hungry for some coherent conceptual models on which to hang my own real-life experiences.

The management literature offers not one but several dozen different conceptual frameworks for looking at change – leaving the non-expert confused about where to start. It was my attempt to make sense of this multiplicity of theories that led me to write a series of six articles published a few years ago in the *British Journal of General Practice* entitled 'Theories of change'. In these articles, I explored six different models of professional and organisational change in relation to effective clinical practice [39–44]:

1. *Adult learning theory*: the notion that adults learn via a cycle of thinking and doing explains why instructional education is so consistently ineffective, and why hands-on practical experience with the opportunity to reflect and discuss with colleagues is the fundamental basis for both learning and change.

2. *Psychoanalytic theory*: Freud's famous concept of the unconscious, which influences (and sometimes overrides) our conscious, rational self. People's resistance to change can sometimes have powerful and deep-rooted emotional explanations.

3. *Group relations theory*: based on studies by specialists at London's Tavistock clinic on how teams operate (or fail to operate) in the work environment. Relationships both within the team and between the team and its wider environment can act as barriers to (or catalysts of) change.

4. *Anthropological theory*: the notion that organisations have cultures – that is, ways of doing things and of thinking about problems – that are, in general, highly resistant to change. A relatively minor proposed change towards evidence-based practice (such as requiring consultants to look up evidence routinely on the Cochrane database) may in reality be highly threatening to the culture of the organisation (in which, for example, the 'consultant opinion' has traditionally carried an almost priestly status).

5. *Classical management theory*: the notion that 'mainstreaming' a change within an organisation requires a systematic plan to make it happen. The vision for change must be shared amongst a critical mass of staff, and must be accompanied by planned changes to the visible structures of the organisation, to the roles and responsibilities of key individuals, and to information and communication systems.

6. *Complexity theory*: the notion that large organisations (such as the UK National Health Service) depend critically on the dynamic, evolving, and local relationships and communication systems between individuals. Supporting key interpersonal relationships, and improving the quality and timeliness of information available locally are often more crucial factors

in achieving sustained change than 'top-down' directives or overarching national or regional programmes.

There are, as I have said, many additional models of change that might come in useful when identifying and overcoming barriers to achieving evidence-based practice. The above-mentioned list is not intended to be exhaustive – and given the complex nature of health care organisations, none of them will provide a simple formula for successful change.

I would certainly add a seventh theoretical model to the list – that of change as a *social movement* – that is, as a powerful groundswell of activity that is bound up with individuals' identity as part of the movement for change [45]. If you've ever been on a protest march, or joined a residents' initiative to improve some local service or other, you'll know what it feels like to be part of a social movement. I was once on a high-level committee that tried to close the little-used casualty department of a small hospital on the grounds that there was no evidence that it was either effective or cost-effective – but I bargained without the input of the 'Hands Off Our Hospital' campaign. Indeed, many successful changes in clinical practice towards evidence-based care (e.g. the abolition of routine episiotomy in obstetric care) were achieved primarily through patient pressure groups operating in 'social movement' mode.

The interesting thing about social movements for change is that as Bate and colleagues [45] emphasise, while they can achieve profound and widespread change, they cannot be planned, controlled or their behaviour predicted in the same way as a conventional management model. You might also like to check out Pope's [46] sociological analysis of the rise of EBM as a social movement!

Whatever theoretical approach you take to change, converting your theories into practice will be a tough challenge. A publication by the UK National Association of Health Authorities and Trusts (NAHAT), entitled 'Acting on the Evidence', emphasises that the task of supporting and empowering managers and clinical professionals to use evidence as part of their everyday decision making is massive and complex [47]. An action checklist for health care organisations working towards an evidence-based culture for clinical and policymaking decisions, listed at the end of Appendix 1, is adapted from the NAHAT report.

First and foremost, key players within the organisation, particularly chief executives, board members and senior clinicians, must create an evidence-based culture where decision-making is *expected* to be based on the best available evidence. High-quality, up-to-date information sources (such as the Cochrane electronic library and the Medline database) should be available in every office, and staff given protected time to access them. Ideally, users should only have to deal with a single access point for all available sources.

Information on the clinical and cost-effectiveness of particular technologies should be produced, disseminated and used together. Individuals who collate and disseminate this information within the organisation need to be aware of who will use it and how it will be applied – and tailor their presentation accordingly. They should also set standards for, and evaluate, the quality of the evidence they are circulating. Individuals on the organisation's internal mailing list for effectiveness information need training and support if they are to make the best use of this information.

This sound advice from NAHAT is based (implicitly if not explicitly) on the notion of the *learning organisation*. As Davies and Nutley [48] have pointed out, 'Learning is something achieved by individuals, but "learning organisations" can configure themselves to maximise, mobilise, and retain this learning potential'. Drawing on the work of Senge [49], they offer five key features of a learning organisation.

1. People are encouraged to move beyond traditional, professional or departmental boundaries (an approach Senge called 'open systems thinking').
2. Individuals' personal learning needs are systematically identified and addressed.
3. Learning occurs to some extent in teams, because it is largely through teams that organisations achieve their objectives.
4. Efforts are made to change the way people conceptualise issues – thus allowing new, creative approaches to old problems.
5. Senior clinicians and managers provide leadership to drive through a shared vision with coherent values and clear strategic direction, so that staff willingly pull together towards a common goal.

Turning a traditional organisation into a learning organisation is a tough task, which often involves a major shift in organisational culture (the unwritten rules, assumptions and expectations that make up 'how things are done around here'). Whilst it's not possible for any single individual to turn an organisation around, if you're sufficiently senior to write the job description of a new member of staff, or to decide how a training budget is spent, or to choose who is involved in a key decision, you can start to move your organisation in the right direction (Table 15.2).

A core principle in developing a learning organisation is *invest in people*. In addition to strong leadership form the top, there are some particular roles that you might think of supporting in relation to EBM [25].

1. *Knowledge managers*: These are senior people hired not just to get the information systems right but to encourage the rest of us to use them. They make the decisions about what software licences to purchase for the organisation and which members of staff are allowed to access which knowledge sources. When I wrote the first edition of this book in 1995, a minority of

Table 15.2 Key differences between a traditional organisation and a learning organisation

Feature	Traditional organisation	Learning organisation
Organisational boundaries	Clearly demarcated	Permeable
Structure of the organisation	Predesigned and fixed	Evolving
Approach to human resources	Minimum skill set to do the job	Maximise skills to enhance creativity and learning
Approach to complex activities	Divide into segmented tasks	Ensure integrated processes
Divisions and departments	Functional, hierarchical groupings	Open, multifunctional networks

Source: Senge [49]. Reproduced with permission of Emerald Group Publishing Limited.

hospitals had a rule that staff nurses couldn't go into the medical library or dial up an Internet connection. The role of the knowledge manager is to blow this sort of nonsense away and ensure that (in the case of EBM) everyone who needs to practice it has links to the relevant knowledge base, protected time to access it and appropriate training.

2. *Knowledge workers*: These individuals have it on their job description to help the rest of us find and apply knowledge. The person on the computer helpdesk is a kind of knowledge worker, as is a librarian or a research assistant. To use some contemporary jargon, the tools of EBM should be offered as an 'augmented product' with designated members of staff hired to provide flexible support to individuals as and when they ask for it.

3. *Champions*: Adoption of a new practice by individuals in an organisation or professional group is more likely if key individuals within that group are willing to back the innovation. 'Backing' an evidence-based innovation might include, for example, talking enthusiastically about it, showing people how to use it, getting it on the agenda of key committees, giving staff protected time to learn about it and try it out, and rewarding people who take it up. Whilst there's remarkably little research evidence about what champions actually do (or what's the most effective way of championing an evidence-based change), the principle is pretty simple: designate particular individuals at every level in your organisation to back it.

4. *Boundary spanners*: An organisation is more likely to adopt a new approach to practice if individuals can be identified who have significant social ties both within and outside the organisation, and who are able and willing to link the organisation to the outside world in relation to this particular practice. Such individuals play a pivotal role in capturing the

ideas that will become organisational innovations. If you've got a member of staff who is well connected in relation to an aspect of evidence-based practice, make a point of drawing on their connections and expertise. Send staff out of the organisation – on conferences, visits to comparable organisations, or to quality improvement collaboratives – and when they return, capture what they have learnt by making time to listen to their stories and ideas.

A specific tool to consider when working towards the 'evidence-based organisation' is the idea of integrated care pathways, defined as pre-defined plans of patient care relating to a specific diagnosis (e.g. suspected fractured hip) or intervention (e.g. hernia repair), with the aim of making the management more structured, consistent and efficient [50]. I have included an example of an attempt to introduce such a pathway in section 'Ten questions to ask about a paper describing a quality improvement initiative'. A good care pathway integrates evidence-based recommendations with the realities of local services, usually via a multi-professional initiative that engages both clinicians and managers. The care pathway states not only what intervention is recommended at different stages in the course of the condition but also whose responsibility it is to undertake the task and to follow up if it gets missed. Whilst there are many care pathways in circulation, it is often the process of developing the pathway as much as the finished product that engages staff across the organisation to focus on evidence-based care in the target condition. If your organisation is resistant to the whole concept of EBM, you might find that the process of developing one care pathway for a relatively uncontroversial condition builds a surprising amount of goodwill and buy-in to the principle of evidence-based practice, which can be drawn upon in rolling out the idea more widely.

Finally, note that the UK National Institute for Health Research Health Service and Delivery Research Programme (see http://www.netscc.ac.uk/hsdr/) is funding an exciting collection of empirical studies on the development, delivery and organisation of health services, many of them highly relevant to the implementation of best practice at the organisational level. There are now over 300 reports of research studies on the implementation of evidence that you can download free of charge.

References

1 Van Someren V. *Changing clinical practice in the light of the evidence: two contrasting stories from perinatology. Getting research findings into practice.* London: BMJ Publications, 1994.

2 Gilstrap LC, Christensen R, Clewell WH, et al. Effect of corticosteroids for fetal maturation on perinatal outcomes. NIH consensus development panel on the effect

of corticosteroids for fetal maturation on perinatal outcomes. JAMA: The Journal of the American Medical Association 1995;**273**(5):413–8.

3 Crowley PA. Antenatal corticosteroid therapy: a meta-analysis of the randomized trials, 1972 to 1994. American Journal of Obstetrics and Gynecology 1995; **173**(1):322–35.

4 Halliday H. Overview of clinical trials comparing natural and synthetic surfactants. Neonatology 1995;**67**(Suppl. 1):32–47.

5 Booth-Clibborn N, Packer C, Stevens A. Health technology diffusion rates. International Journal of Technology Assessment in Health Care 2000;**16**(3):781–6.

6 Chauhan D, Mason A. Factors affecting the uptake of new medicines in secondary care–a literature review. Journal of Clinical Pharmacy and Therapeutics 2008;**33**(4):339–48.

7 Garjón FJ, Azparren A, Vergara I, et al. Adoption of new drugs by physicians: a survival analysis. BMC Health Services Research 2012;**12**(1):56.

8 Robert G, Greenhalgh T, MacFarlane F, et al. Organisational factors influencing technology adoption and assimilation in the NHS: a systematic literature review. Report for the National Institute for Health Research Service Delivery and Organisation programme, London, 2009.

9 Woolf SH, Johnson RE. The break-even point: when medical advances are less important than improving the fidelity with which they are delivered. The Annals of Family Medicine 2005;**3**(6):545–52.

10 Caulford PG, Lamb SB, Kaigas TB, et al. Physician incompetence: specific problems and predictors. Academic Medicine 1994;**69**(10):S16–8.

11 Michie S, Johnston M, Francis J, et al. From theory to intervention: mapping theoretically derived behavioural determinants to behaviour change techniques. Applied Psychology 2008;**57**(4):660–80.

12 Eccles M, Grimshaw J, Walker A, et al. Changing the behavior of healthcare professionals: the use of theory in promoting the uptake of research findings. Journal of Clinical Epidemiology 2005;**58**(2):107–12.

13 Horsley T, Hyde C, Santesso N, et al. Teaching critical appraisal skills in healthcare settings. Cochrane Database of Systematic Reviews. The Cochrane Library 2011;(05): 2001;(3):CD001270.

14 Taylor R, Reeves B, Ewings P, et al. A systematic review of the effectiveness of critical appraisal skills training for clinicians. Medical Education 2000;**34**(2):120–5.

15 Coomarasamy A, Khan KS. What is the evidence that postgraduate teaching in evidence based medicine changes anything? A systematic review. BMJ: British Medical Journal 2004;**329**(7473):1017.

16 Norman GR, Shannon SI. Effectiveness of instruction in critical appraisal (evidence-based medicine) skills: a critical appraisal. Canadian Medical Association Journal 1998;**158**(2):177–81.

17 Green ML. Evidence-based medicine training in internal medicine residency programs. Journal of General Internal Medicine 2000;**15**(2):129–33.

18 Green ML. Evidence-based medicine training in graduate medical education: past, present and future. Journal of Evaluation in Clinical Practice 2000;**6**(2):121–38.

19 Green ML, Ruff TR. Why do residents fail to answer their clinical questions? A qualitative study of barriers to practicing evidence-based medicine. Academic Medicine 2005;**80**(2):176–82.

20 Grimshaw J, Thomas R, MacLennan G, et al. Effectiveness and efficiency of guideline dissemination and implementation strategies. Health Technology Assessment 2004;**8**:1–72.

21 Giguère A, Légaré F, Grimshaw J, et al. Printed educational materials: effects on professional practice and healthcare outcomes. Cochrane Database of Systematic Reviews 2012;**10**.

22 Hysong SJ. Meta-analysis: audit and feedback features impact effectiveness on care quality. Medical Care 2009;**47**(3):356–63.

23 Flodgren G, Eccles MP, Shepperd S, et al. An overview of reviews evaluating the effectiveness of financial incentives in changing healthcare professional behaviours and patient outcomes. Cochrane Database of Systematic Reviews (Online) 2011;7.

24 Scott A, Sivey P, Ait Ouakrim D, et al. The effect of financial incentives on the quality of health care provided by primary care physicians. Cochrane Database of Systematic Reviews (Online) 2011;**9**.

25 Greenhalgh T, Robert G, Macfarlane F, et al. Diffusion of innovations in service organizations: systematic review and recommendations. Milbank Quarterly 2004;**82**(4):581–629.

26 Rogers E. *Diffusion of innovations, 4th edition.* New York: Simon and Schuster, 2010.

27 Locock L, Dopson S, Chambers D, et al. Understanding the role of opinion leaders in improving clinical effectiveness. Social Science & Medicine 2001;**53**(6):745–57.

28 Flodgren G, Parmelli E, Doumit G, et al. Local opinion leaders: effects on professional practice and health care outcomes. Cochrane Database of Systematic Reviews (Online) 2011;**8**.

29 Fischer MA, Avorn J. Academic detailing can play a key role in assessing and implementing comparative effectiveness research findings. Health Affairs 2012;**31**(10):2206–12.

30 Garg AX, Adhikari NK, McDonald H, et al. Effects of computerized clinical decision support systems on practitioner performance and patient outcomes. JAMA: The Journal of the American Medical Association 2005;**293**(10):1223–38.

31 Black AD, Car J, Pagliari C, et al. The impact of eHealth on the quality and safety of health care: a systematic overview. PLoS Medicine 2011;**8**(1):e1000387.

32 Wong G, Greenhalgh T, Westhorp G, et al. RAMESES publication standards: realist syntheses. BMC Medicine 2013;**11**:21 doi: 10.1186/1741-7015-11-21[published Online First: Epub Date].

33 Zahra SA, George G. Absorptive capacity: a review, reconceptualization, and extension. Academy of Management Review 2002;**27**(2):185–203.

34 Ferlie E, Gabbay J, Fitzgerald L, et al. Evidence-based medicine and organisational change: an overview of some recent qualitative research, 2001.

35 Dopson S, FitzGerald L, Ferlie E, et al. No magic targets! Changing clinical practice to become more evidence based. Health Care Management Review 2010;**35**(1):2–12.

36 Pettigrew AM, Ferlie E, McKee L. *Shaping strategic change: making change in large organizations: the case of the National Health Service.* London: Sage, 1992.

37 Gustafson DH, Sainfort F, Eichler M, et al. Developing and testing a model to predict outcomes of organizational change. Health Services Research 2003; **38**(2):751–76.

38 Ferlie E, Crilly T, Jashapara A, et al. Knowledge mobilisation in healthcare: a critical review of health sector and generic management literature. Social Science & Medicine 2012;**74**(8):1297–304.

39 Greenhalgh T. Change and the team: group relations theory. British Journal of General Practice 2000;**50**:262–63.

40 Greenhalgh T. Change and the organisation 2: strategy. British Journal of General Practice 2000;**50**:424–5.

41 Greenhalgh T. Change and the organisation 1: culture and context. British Journal of General Practice 2000;**50**:340–1.

42 Greenhalgh T. Change and the individual 2: psychoanalytic theory. British Journal of General Practice 2000;**50**:164–5.

43 Greenhalgh T. Change and the individual 1: adult learning theory. British Journal of General Practice 2000;**50**:76–7.

44 Greenhalgh T. Change and complexity: the rich picture. British Journal of General Practice 2000:514–5.

45 Bate P, Robert G, Bevan H. The next phase of healthcare improvement: what can we learn from social movements? Quality and Safety in Health Care 2004;**13**(1):62–6.

46 Pope C. Resisting evidence: the study of evidence-based medicine as a contemporary social movement. Health 2003;**7**(3):267–82.

47 Appleby J, Walshe K, Ham C, et al. Acting on the evidence: a review of clinical effectiveness – sources of information, dissemination and implementation. NHS Confederation, Leeds, 1995.

48 Davies HT, Nutley SM. Developing learning organisations in the new NHS. BMJ: British Medical Journal 2000;**320**(7240):998.

49 Senge PM. The fifth discipline. Measuring Business Excellence 1997;**1**(3):46–51.

50 Rotter T, Kinsman L, James E, et al. Clinical pathways: effects on professional practice, patient outcomes, length of stay and hospital costs. Cochrane Database of Systematic Reviews (Online) 2010;**3**(3).

Chapter 16 Applying evidence with patients

The patient perspective

There is no such thing as *the* patient perspective – and that is precisely the point of this chapter. At times in our lives, often more frequently the older we get, we are all patients. Some of us are also health professionals – but when the decision relates to *our* health, *our* medication, *our* operation, the side effects that *we* may or may not experience with a particular treatment, we look on that decision differently from when we make the same kind of decision in our professional role.

As you will know by now if you have read the earlier chapters of this book, evidence-based medicine (EBM) is mainly about using some kind of population average – an odds ratio, a number needed to treat, an estimate of mean effect size, and so on – to inform decisions. But very few of us will behave exactly like the point average on the graph: some will be more susceptible to benefit and some more susceptible to harm from a particular intervention. And few of us will value a particular outcome to the same extent as a group average on (say) a standard gamble question (see section 'How can we help ensure that evidence-based guidelines are followed?').

The individual unique experience of being ill (or indeed being 'at risk' or classified as such) can be expressed in narrative terms: that is, a story can be told about it. And everyone's story is different. The 'same' set of symptoms or piece of news will have a host of different meanings depending on who is experiencing them and what else is going on in their lives. The exercise of taking a history from a patient is an attempt to 'tame' this individual, idiosyncratic set of personal experiences and put it into a more or less standard format to align with the protocols for assessing, treating and preventing disease. Indeed, England's first professor of general practice, Marshall Marinker [1],

How to Read a Paper: The Basics of Evidence-Based Medicine, Fifth Edition. Trisha Greenhalgh. © 2014 John Wiley & Sons, Ltd. Published 2014 by John Wiley & Sons, Ltd.

once said that the role of medicine is to distinguish the clear message of the disease from the interfering noise of the patient as a person.

As I have written elsewhere, an EBM perspective on *disease* and the patient's unique perspective on his or her *illness* ('narrative-based medicine', if you like) are not at all incompatible [2].

It is worth going back to the original definition of EBM proposed by Sackett and colleagues. This definition is reproduced in full, although only the first sentence is generally quoted.

> *Evidence based medicine is the conscientious, explicit, and judicious use of current best evidence in making decisions about the care of individual patients. The practice of evidence based medicine means integrating individual clinical expertise with the best available external clinical evidence from systematic research. By individual clinical expertise we mean the proficiency and judgment that individual clinicians acquire through clinical experience and clinical practice. Increased expertise is reflected in many ways, but especially in more effective and efficient diagnosis and in the more thoughtful identification and compassionate use of individual patients' predicaments, rights, and preferences in making clinical decisions about their care. By best available external clinical evidence we mean clinically relevant research, often from the basic sciences of medicine, but especially from patient centred clinical research into the accuracy and precision of diagnostic tests (including the clinical examination), the power of prognostic markers, and the efficacy and safety of therapeutic, rehabilitative, and preventive regimens (p. 71).*

Thus, while the original protagonists of EBM are sometimes wrongly depicted as having airbrushed the poor patient out of the script, they were actually very careful to depict EBM as being contingent on patient choice (and, incidentally, as dependent on clinical judgement). The 'best' treatment is not necessarily the one shown to be most efficacious in randomised controlled trials but the one that fits a particular set of individual circumstances and aligns with the patient's preferences and priorities.

The 'evidence-based' approach is sometimes stereotypically depicted by the clinician who feels, for example, that every patient with a transient ischaemic attack should take warfarin because this is the most efficacious preventive therapy, whether or not the patients say they don't want to take tablets, can't face the side effects or feel that attending for a blood test every week to check their clotting function is not worth the hassle. A relative of mine was reluctant to take warfarin, for example, because she had been advised to stop eating grapefruit – a food she has enjoyed for breakfast for over 60 years but which contains chemicals that may interact with warfarin. I was pleased that her general practitioner (GP) invited her to come in and discuss the pros and cons of the different treatment options, so that her choice would an informed one.

Almost all research in the EBM tradition between 1990 and 2010 focused on the epidemiological component and sought to build an evidence base of randomised controlled trials and other 'methodologically robust' research designs. Later, a tradition of 'evidence-based patient choice' emerged in which the patient's right to choose the option most appropriate and acceptable to them was formalised and systematically studied [3]. The third component of EBM referred to in the quote – individual clinical judgement – has not been extensively theorised by scholars within the EBM tradition, although I have written about it myself [4].

PROMs

Before we get into how to involve patients in individualising the decisions of EBM, I want to introduce a relatively new approach to selecting the outcome measures used in clinical trials: patient-reported outcome measures or PROMs. Here's a definition.

> *PROM's are the tools we use to gain insight from the perspective of the patient into how aspects of their health and the impact the disease and its treatment are perceived to be having on their lifestyle and subsequently their quality of life (QoL). They are typically self-completed questionnaires, which can be completed by a patient or individual about themselves, or by others on their behalf* [5].

By 'outcome measure' I mean the aspect of health or illness that researchers choose to measure to demonstrate (say) whether a treatment has been effective. Death is an outcome measure. So is blood pressure. So is the chance of leaving hospital with a live baby when you go into hospital in labour. So is the ability to walk upstairs or make a cup of tea on your own. I could go on – but the point is that in any study the researchers have to define what it is they are trying to influence.

PROMs are not individualised measures. On the contrary, they are still a form of population average, but unlike most outcome measures, they are an average of what matters most to patients rather than an average of what researchers or clinicians felt they ought to measure. The way to develop a PROM is to undertake an extensive phase of qualitative research (see Chapter 12) with a representative sample of people who have the condition you are interested in, analyse the qualitative data and then use it to design a survey instrument ('questionnaire', see Chapter 13) that captures all the key features of what patients are concerned about [6, 7].

PROMs were (I believe) first popularised by a team in Oxford led by Ray Fitzpatrick, who used the concept to develop measures for assessing the success of hip and knee replacement surgery [8]. They are now used fairly routinely in many clinical topics in the wider field of 'outcomes research' [9, 10]; and a recent monograph by the UK Kings Fund recommends their routine use in National Health Service decision-making [11]. Just as this edition went to press, the *Journal of the American Medical Association* published a set of standards for PROMs [12].

Shared decision-making

Important though PROMs are, they only tell us what patients, on average, value most, not what the patient in front of us values most. To find that out, as I said back in Chapter 1, you would have to ask the patient. And there is now a science and a methodology for 'asking the patient' [3, 13].

The science of shared decision-making began in the late 1990s as a quirky interest of some keen academic GPs, notably Elwyn and Edwards [14]. The idea is based on the notion of the patient as a rational chooser, able and willing (perhaps with support) to join in the deliberation over options and make an informed choice.

One challenge is maintaining equipoise – that is, holding back on what you feel the course of action should be and setting out the different options with the pros and cons presented objectively, so the patients can make their own decision [15]. Box 16.1 lists the competencies that clinicians need to practise shared decision-making with their patients [16].

Box 16.1 Competencies for shared decision-making (see reference [14])

Define the problem – clear specification of the problem that requires a decision.

Portray equipoise – that professionals may not have a clear preference about which treatment option is the best in the context.

Portray options – one or more treatment options and the option of no treatment if relevant.

Provide information in preferred format – identify patients' preferences if they are to be useful to the decision-making process.

Check understanding – of the range of options and information provided about them.

Explore ideas, concerns and expectations about the clinical condition, possible treatment options and outcomes.

Checking role preference – that patients accept the process and identify their decision-making role preference.

Decision-making – involving the patient to the extent they desire to be involved.

Deferment if necessary – reviewing treatment needs and preferences after time for further consideration, including with friends or family members, if the patient requires.

Review arrangements – a specified time period to review the decision.

The various instruments and tools to support shared decision-making have evolved over the years. At the very least, a decision aid would have a way of making the rather dry information of EBM more accessible to a non-expert, for example by turning numerical data into diagrams and pictures [17]. An example, shown in Figure 16.1, uses colours and simple icons to convey

1. What is my risk of having a heart attack in the next 10 years?

The risk for 100 people like you who DO NOT take statins

NO STATIN
80 people DO NOT have a heart attack (grey, happy)

20 people DO have a heart attack (grey, sad)

The risk for 100 people like you who DO take statins

YES STATIN
80 people still DO NOT have a heart attack (grey, happy)

5 people AVOIDED heart attack (white, happy)

15 people still DO have a heart attack (grey, sad)

95 people experienced NO BENEFIT from taking statins

🙂 Had a heart attack
🙂 Avoided a heart attack
🙂 Didn't have a heart attack

2. What are the downsides of taking statins (cholesterol pill)?

• Statins need to be taken every day for a long time (maybe forever)
• Statins cost money (to you or your drug plan)
• Common side effects: nausea, diarrhoea, constipation (most patients can tolerate)
• Muscle aching/stiffness: 5 in 100 patients (some need to stop statins because of this)
• Liver blood test goes up (no pain, no permanent liver damage): 2 in 100 patients (some need to stop statins because of this)
• Muscle and kidney damage: 1 in 20 000 patients requires patients to stop statins

3. What do you want to do now?

☐ Take (or continue to take) statins

☐ Not take (or stop taking) statins

☐ Prefer to decide at some other time

Figure 16.1 Example of a decision aid: choosing statin in a diabetes patient with a 20% risk of myocardial infarction. Source: Reproduced from reference 18.

quantitative estimates of risk [18]. The ways of measuring the extent to which patients have been involved in a decision have also evolved [19].

Coulter and Collins [20] have produced an excellent guide called *Making Shared Decision-Making a Reality*, which sets out the characteristics of a really good decision aid (Box 16.2).

Increasingly commonly, decision aids are available online, allowing the patient to click through different steps in the decision algorithm (with or without support from a health professional). In my view, the best way to get your head round shared decision-making tools is to take a look at a few – and if possible, put them to use in practice. The UK National Health Service has a website with links to tools for sharing decisions, from abdominal aortic aneurysm repair to stroke prevention in atrial fibrillation: see http://sdm.rightcare.nhs.uk/pda/. A similar (and more comprehensive) range of decision tools is available from this Canadian site: http://decisionaid .ohri.ca/AZinvent.php.

Option grids

Studies using the 'OPTION' instrument suggest that patient involvement in evidence-based decision-making is not always as high as the idealists would

---

Box 16.2 Characteristics of a good decision aid (from reference [17])

Decision aids are different from traditional patient information materials because they do not tell people what to do. Instead, they set out the facts and help people to deliberate about the options. They usually contain:

- a description of the condition and symptoms;
- the likely prognosis with and without treatment;
- the treatment and self-management support options and outcome probabilities;
- what's known from the evidence and not known (uncertainties);
- illustrations to help people understand what it would be like to experience some of the most frequent side effects or complications of the treatment options (often using patient interviews);
- a means of helping people clarify their preferences;
- references and sources of further information;
- the authors' credentials, funding source and declarations of conflict of interest.

like it to be [19]. These days, most health professionals are (allegedly) keen to share decisions with patients in principle, but qualitative and questionnaire research has shown that they perceive a number of barriers to doing so in practice, including time constraints and lack of applicability of the decision support model to the unique predicament of a particular patient [21]. It is relatively uncommon for doctors to refer patients to decision support websites, partly because they feel they are already sharing decisions in routine consultation talk, and partly because they feel that patents do not wish to be involved in this way [22].

The reality of a typical general practice consultation, for example, is a long way from the objective reality of a formal decision algorithm. When a patient attends with symptoms suggestive of (say) sciatica, the doctor has 10 min to make progress. Typically, they will examine the patient, order some tests and then have a rather blurry conversation about how (on the one hand) the patient's symptoms might resolve with physiotherapy but (on the other hand) they might like to see a specialist because some cases will need an operation. The patient typically expresses a vague preference for either conservative or interventionist management, and the doctor (respecting the 'empowered' views) goes along with the patient's preference.

If the doctor is committed to evidence-based shared decision-making, he or she may try using a more structured approach to shared decision-making as set out in section 'Shared decision-making', for example, by logging on to an online algorithm or by using pie charts or pre-programmed spreadsheets to elicit numerical scores of how much the patient values particular procedures and outcomes vis a vis one another. But very often, such tools will have been tried once or twice and then abandoned as technocratic, time-consuming, overly quantitative and oddly disengaged from the unique personal illness narrative that fills the consultation.

The good news is that our colleagues working in the field of shared decision-making have recently acknowledged that the perfect may be the enemy of the good. Most discussions about management options in clinical practice do not require – and may even be thrown off kilter by – an exhaustive analysis of probabilities, risks and preference scores. What most people want is a brief but balanced list of the options, setting out the costs and benefits of each and including an answer to the question 'what would happen if I went down this route?'.

Enter the option grid (http://www.optiongrid.org): the product of a collaborative initiative between patients, doctors and academics [23]. An option grid is a one-page table covering a single topic (so far complete are sciatica, chronic kidney disease, breast cancer, tonsillitis and a dozen or so more). The grid lists the different options as columns, with each row answering a different question (such as 'what does the treatment involve?', 'how soon would I feel better?' and 'how would this treatment affect my ability to work?'). An example is shown in Figure 16.2.

Option grids are developed in a similar way to PROMs, but there is often more of a focus on involvement of the multidisciplinary clinical team, as in this example of an option grid for head and neck cancer management [24]. The distinguishing feature of the option grid approach is that it promotes and supports what has been termed *option talk* – that is, the discussions and deliberations around the different options [25]. The grids are, in effect, analog rather than digital in design.

Sciatica from a slipped (herniated) disc
This grid is designed to help you and your healthcare professional select the treatment option that is best for you. It is for people diagnosed with a herniated disc who have experienced sciatica pain for at least six weeks and is not for people with bowel and urine problems due to the disc pressing on their nerves. Ask your healthcare professional if there are other treatment options available to you.

Frequently asked questions	Managing without Injections or Surgery	Injections (epidural steroids)	Surgery
What does the treatment involve?	Taking pain relievers that reduce inflammation around the nerve and attempting to be as active as possible. Physical therapy may also help.	A needle is used to inject local anaesthetic and steroid where the nerve is under pressure near the spine. An injection is normally performed at a special clinic and takes around 20 minutes.	The slipped disc that puts pressure on the nerve is removed during an operation on the back. The operation takes approximately 2 hours. Most people stay in hospital for a night or two but some go home the day of the surgery.
How soon will I feel better?	6 weeks after diagnosis, roughly 20 in 100 people say they are very or somewhat satisfied with their symptoms.	Most people who experience relief feel better within the first week or so after the injection.	6 weeks after surgery, roughly 60 in 100 people say they are very or somewhat satisfied with their symptoms.
Which treatment gives the best long-term results?	1 year after diagnosis, around 45 in 100 people who manage without surgery or injections say they are very or somewhat satisfied with their symptoms.	It is hard to say: some studies have shown benefits from steroid injections but others have not.	1 year after surgery, around 70 in 100 people say they are very or somewhat satisfied with their symptoms.
What are the main risks/side effects associated with this treatment?	All medications have some side effects. Being active is unlikely to make your sciatica harder to treat in the future.	Fewer than 1 in 100 people have complications, which could potentially include bleeding, headache, and infection.	The main risks associated with this surgery are infection (2 in 100), blood clots (1 in 100) and damage to the nerves (less than 1 in 100).
How will this treatment impact my ability to work?	You should return to your daily activities and return to work as soon as you are able to do so.	Most people return to work and normal activities the day after the injection.	Most people are off work for 6-8 weeks following this operation.
Will I need any other treatment?	Keep active. You may be referred to a physical therapist to start an exercise program.	You should take pain relievers as needed and keep active. The injection may be repeated in the future, usually no more than 2 or 3 times total.	Most people undergo physical therapy after surgery and use pain relievers to manage postoperative pain. In the years after surgery, a small number of people will require more surgery (around 5 in 100 within the first year).

Figure 16.2 Example of an option grid. Source: http://www.optiongrid.org/optiongrids.php. Reproduced with permission of Glyn Elwyn.

The reason I see this approach as progress from more algorithmic approaches to shared decision-making introduced in section 'The patient perspective' is that the information in an option grid is presented in a format that allows both reflection and dialogue. The grid can be printed off (or indeed, the patient can be given the url) and invited to go away and consider the options before returning for a further consultation. And unlike the previous generation of shared decision-making tools, neither the patient nor the clinician needs to be a 'geek' to use them.

n of 1 trials and other individualised approaches

The last approach to involving patients that I want to introduce in this chapter is the *n* of 1 trial. This is a very simple design in which each participant receives, in randomly allocated order, both the intervention and the control treatment.

An example is probably the best way to explain this. Back in 1994, some Australian GPs wanted to address the clinical issue of which painkiller to use in osteoarthritis [26]. Some patients, they felt, did fine on paracetamol (which has relatively few side effects), while others did not respond so well to paracetamol but obtained great relief from a non-steroidal anti-inflammatory drug (NSAID). In the normal clinical setting, one might try paracetamol first and move to the NSAID if the patient did not respond. But supposing there was a strong placebo effect? The patient might conceivably have limited confidence in paracetamol because it is such a commonplace drug, whereas an NSAID in a fancy package might be subconsciously favoured.

The idea of the *n* of 1 trial is that all treatments are anonmyised, prepared in identical formulations and packaging, and just labelled 'A', 'B', and so on. The participants do not know which drug they are taking, hence their response is not influenced by whether they 'believe in' the treatment. To add to scientific rigour, the drugs may be taken in sequence such as ABAB or AABB, with 'washout' periods in between.

March and colleagues' *n* of 1 trial of paracetamol versus NSAIDs did confirm the clinical hunch that some patients did markedly better on the NSAID but many did equally well on paracetamol. Importantly, unlike a standard randomised trial, the *n* of 1 design allowed the researchers to identify which patients were in each category. But the withdrawal rate from the trial was high, partly because when participants found a medication that worked, they just wanted to keep taking it rather than swap to the alternative!

But despite its conceptual elegance and a distant promise of linking to the 'personalised medicine' paradigm in which every patient will have their tests and treatment options individualised to their particular genome, physiome, microbiome, and so on, the n of 1 trial has not caught on widely in either research or clinical practice. A review article by Lillie and colleagues [27] suggests why. Such trials are labour intensive to carry out, requiring a high degree of individual personalisation and large amounts of data for every participant. 'Washout' periods raise practical and ethical problems (does one have to endure one's arthritis with no pain relief for several weeks to serve the scientific endeavour?). Combining the findings from different participants raises statistical challenges. And the (conceptually simple) science of n of 1 trials has begun to get muddled up with the much more complex and uncertain science of personalised medicine.

In short, the n of 1 trial is a useful design (and one you may be asked about in exams!), but it is not the panacea it was once predicted to be.

A recent (and somewhat untested) alternative approach to individualising treatment regimens has been proposed recently by Moore and colleagues [28] in relation to pain relief. Their basic argument is that we should 'expect failure' (because the number needed to treat for many interventions is more than 2, statistically speaking any individual is more likely *not* to benefit than benefit) but 'pursue success' (because the 'average' for any intervention response masks a subgroup of responders who will do very well on that intervention). They propose a process of guided trial and error, systematically trying one intervention followed by another, until the one that works effectively for *this* patient is identified. Perhaps this is the n of 1 trial without worrying either about the placebo element or about the fact that one may need to try half a dozen options before finding the best one in the circumstances.

References

1 Marinker M. The chameleon, the Judas goat, and the cuckoo. The Journal of the Royal College of General Practitioners 1978;**28**(189):199–206.

2 Greenhalgh T. Narrative based medicine: narrative based medicine in an evidence based world. BMJ: British Medical Journal 1999;**318**(7179):323.

3 Edwards A, Elwyn G. *Shared decision-making in health care: achieving evidence-based patient choice*. New York: Oxford University Press, 2009.

4 Greenhalgh T. Uncertainty and clinical method. Clinical Uncertainty in Primary Care: Springer, 2013:23–45.

5 Meadows KA. Patient-reported outcome measures: an overview. British Journal of Community Nursing 2011;**16**(3):146–51.

6 Garratt A, Schmidt L, Mackintosh A, et al. Quality of life measurement: bibliographic study of patient assessed health outcome measures. BMJ: British Medical Journal 2002;**324**(7351):1417.

7 Ader DN. Developing the patient-reported outcomes measurement information system (PROMIS). Medical Care 2007;**45**(5):S1–2.

8 Dawson J, Fitzpatrick R, Murray D, et al. Questionnaire on the perceptions of patients about total knee replacement. Journal of Bone & Joint Surgery, British Volume 1998;**80**(1):63–9.

9 Dawson J, Doll H, Fitzpatrick R, et al. The routine use of patient reported outcome measures in healthcare settings. BMJ: British Medical Journal (Clinical Research ed.) 2009;**340**:c186.

10 McGrail K, Bryan S, Davis J. Let's all go to the PROM: the case for routine patient-reported outcome measurement in Canadian healthcare. HealthcarePapers 2011;**11**(4):8–18.

11 Devlin NJ, Appleby J, Buxton M. *Getting the most out of PROMs: putting health outcomes at the heart of NHS decision-making*. King's Fund, London, 2010.

12 Basch E. Standards for patient-reported outcome-based performance measures standards for patient-reported outcome-based performance measures viewpoint. JAMA: The Journal of Medical Association 2013;**310**(2):139–40 doi: 10.1001/jama.2013.6855[published Online First: Epub Date]|.

13 Makoul G, Clayman ML. An integrative model of shared decision making in medical encounters. Patient Education and Counseling 2006;**60**(3):301–12.

14 Elwyn G, Edwards A, Kinnersley P. Shared decision-making in primary care: the neglected second half of the consultation. The British Journal of General Practice 1999;**49**(443):477–82.

15 Elwyn G, Edwards A, Kinnersley P, et al. Shared decision making and the concept of equipoise: the competences of involving patients in healthcare choices. The British Journal of General Practice 2000;**50**(460):892–9.

16 Edwards A, Elwyn G, Hood K, et al. Patient-based outcome results from a cluster randomized trial of shared decision making skill development and use of risk communication aids in general practice. Family Practice 2004;**21**(4):347–54.

17 Edwards A, Elwyn G, Mulley A. Explaining risks: turning numerical data into meaningful pictures. BMJ: British Medical Journal 2002;**324**(7341):827.

18 Stiggelbout A, Weijden T, Wit MD, et al. Shared decision making: really putting patients at the centre of healthcare. BMJ: British Medical Journal 2012;**344**:e256.

19 Elwyn G, Hutchings H, Edwards A, et al. The OPTION scale: measuring the extent that clinicians involve patients in decision-making tasks. Health Expectations 2005;**8**(1):34–42.

20 Coulter A, Collins A. *Making shared decision-making a reality. No decision about me, without me*. The King's Fund, London, 2011.

21 Gravel K, Légaré F, Graham ID. Barriers and facilitators to implementing shared decision-making in clinical practice: a systematic review of health professionals' perceptions. Implementation Science 2006;**1**(1):16.

22 Elwyn G, Rix A, Holt T, et al. Why do clinicians not refer patients to online decision support tools? Interviews with front line clinics in the NHS. BMJ Open 2012;**2**(6) doi: 10.1136/bmjopen-2012-001530[published Online First: Epub Date]|.

23 Elwyn G, Lloyd A, Joseph-Williams N, et al. Option Grids: shared decision making made easier. Patient Education and Counseling 2013;**90**:207–12.

24 Elwyn G, Lloyd A, Williams NJ, et al. Shared decision-making in a multidisciplinary head and neck cancer team: a case study of developing Option Grids. International Journal of Person Centered Medicine 2012;**2**(3):421–6.

25 Thomson R, Kinnersley P, Barry M. Shared decision making: a model for clinical practice. Journal of General Internal Medicine 2012;**27**(10):1361–7.
26 March L, Irwig L, Schwarz J, et al. n of 1 trials comparing a non-steroidal anti-inflammatory drug with paracetamol in osteoarthritis. BMJ: British Medical Journal 1994;**309**(6961):1041–6.
27 Lillie EO, Patay B, Diamant J, et al. The n-of-1 clinical trial: the ultimate strategy for individualizing medicine? Personalized Medicine 2011;**8**(2):161–73.
28 Moore A, Derry S, Eccleston C, et al. Expect analgesic failure; pursue analgesic success. BMJ: British Medical Journal 2013;**346**:f2690.

Chapter 17 Criticisms of evidence-based medicine

What's wrong with EBM when it's done badly?

This new chapter is necessary because evidence-based medicine (EBM) has long outlived its honeymoon period. There is, quite appropriately, a growing body of scholarship that offers legitimate criticisms of EBM's assumptions and core approaches. There is also a somewhat larger body of misinformed critique – and a grey zone of 'anti-EBM' writing that contains more than a grain of truth but is itself one-sided and poorly argued. This chapter seeks to set out the legitimate criticisms and point the interested reader towards more in-depth arguments.

To inform this chapter, I have drawn on a number of sources: a widely cited short article by BMJ columnist and common-sense general practitioner (GP), Spence [1]; a book by Timmermans and Berg [2] called *The Gold Standard: The challenge of evidence-based medicine and standardization in health care*; a paper by Timmermans and Mauck [3] on the promises and pitfalls of EBM; a '20 years on' reflection by some EBM gurus [4]; Goldacre's [5] book 'Bad Pharma'; and some additional materials on evidence-based policymaking referenced in Section 'Why is 'evidence-based policymaking' so hard to achieve?'.

The first thing we need to get clear is the distinction between EBM when it is practised badly (this section) and EBM when it is practised well (next section). As a starter for this section, I am going to reproduce two paragraphs from the preface to this book, written for the first edition way back in 1995 and still unchanged in this fifth edition:

Many of the descriptions given by cynics of what evidence-based medicine is (the glorification of things that can be measured without regard for the usefulness or accuracy of what is measured, the uncritical

How to Read a Paper: The Basics of Evidence-Based Medicine, Fifth Edition. Trisha Greenhalgh.
© 2014 John Wiley & Sons, Ltd. Published 2014 by John Wiley & Sons, Ltd.

acceptance of published numerical data, the preparation of
all-encompassing guidelines by self-appointed 'experts' who are out of
touch with real medicine, the debasement of clinical freedom through
the imposition of rigid and dogmatic clinical protocols, and the
over-reliance on simplistic, inappropriate, and often incorrect economic
analyses) are actually criticisms of what the evidence-based medicine
movement is fighting against, rather than of what it represents.

Do not, however, think of me as an evangelist for the gospel according to
evidence-based medicine. I believe that the science of finding, evaluating
and implementing the results of medical research can, and often does,
make patient care more objective, more logical, and more cost-effective.
If I didn't believe that, I wouldn't spend so much of my time teaching it
and trying, as a general practitioner, to practise it. Nevertheless, I
believe that when applied in a vacuum (that is, in the absence of
common sense and without regard to the individual circumstances and
priorities of the person being offered treatment or to the complex nature
of clinical practice and policymaking), 'evidence-based' decision-making
is a reductionist process with a real potential for harm.

Let's unpack these issues further. What does 'EBM practised badly' look like?

First, bad EBM cites numbers derived from population studies but asks no upstream questions about where those numbers (or studies) came from. If you have spent time on the wards or in general practice, you will know the type of person who tends to do this: a fast-talking, technically adept individual who appears to know the literature and how to access it (perhaps via apps on their state-of-the-art tablet computer), and who always seems to have an NNT (number needed to treat) or odds ratio at his or her fingertips. But the fast talker is less skilled at justifying why *this* set of 'evidence-based' figures should be privileged over some other set of figures. Their evidence, for example, may come from a single trial rather than a high-quality and recent meta-analysis of all available trials. Self-appointed fast-talking EBM 'experts' tend to be unreflective (i.e. they don't spend much time thinking deeply about things) and they rarely engage *critically* with the numbers they are citing. They may not, for example, have engaged with the arguments about surrogate endpoints I set out on page 81.

Bad EBM considers the world of published evidence to equate to the world of patient need. Hence, it commits two fallacies: it assumes that if (say) a randomised controlled trial (RCT) exists that tested a treatment for a 'disease', that disease is necessarily a real medical problem requiring treatment;

and it also assumes that if 'methodologically robust' evidence does not exist on a topic, that topic is unimportant. This leads to a significant bias. The evidence base will accumulate in conditions that offer the promise of profit to the pharmaceutical and medical device industries – such as the detection, monitoring and management of risk factors for cardiovascular disease [6]; the development and testing of new drug entities for diabetes [7], or the creation and treatment of non-diseases such as 'female hypoactive sexual desire' [8]). Evidence will also accumulate in conditions that government chooses to recognise and prioritise for publicly funded research, but it will fail to accumulate (or will accumulate much more slowly) in Cinderella conditions that industry and/or government deem unimportant, hard-to-classify or 'non-medical', such as multi-morbidity [9], physical activity in cardiovascular prevention [10], domestic violence [11] or age-related frailty [12].

Bad EBM has little regard for the patient perspective and fails to acknowledge the significance of clinical judgement. As I pointed out in Section 'The patient perspective', the 'best' treatment is not necessarily the one shown to be most efficacious in RCTs but the one that fits a particular set of individual circumstances and aligns with the patient's preferences and priorities.

Finally, bad EBM draws on bad research – for example, research that has used weak sampling strategies, unjustified sample sizes, inappropriate comparators, statistical trick-cycling, and so on. Chapter 6 set out some specific ways in which research (and the way it is presented) can mislead. Whilst people behaving in this way will often claim to be members of the EBM community (e.g. their papers may have 'evidence-based' in the title), the more scholarly members of that community would strongly dispute such claims.

What's wrong with EBM when it's done well?

Whilst I worry as a clinician about EBM done badly, the academic in me is more interested in its limitations when done well. This is because there are good philosophical reasons why EBM will never be the fount of all knowledge.

A significant criticism of EBM, highlighted by Timmermans and Berg in their book, is the extent to which EBM is a formalised method for imposing an unjustifiable degree of standardisation and control over clinical practice. They argue that in the modern clinical world, EBM can be more or less equated with the production and implementation of clinical practice guidelines. 'Yet', they argue (p. 3), 'such evidence is only rarely available to cover all the decision moments of a guideline. To fill in the blanks and to interpret conflicting statements that might exist in the literature, additional, less objective steps [such as consensus methods] are necessary to create a guideline' [2].

Because of these (sometimes subtle) gaps in the research base, Timmermans and Berg contend that an 'evidence-based' guideline is usually not nearly as evidence-based as it appears to be. But the *formalisation* of the evidence into guidelines, which may then become ossified in protocols or computerised decision support programmes, lends an unjustified level of significance – and sometimes coercion – to the guideline. The rough edges are sanded down, the holes are filled in and the resulting recommendations start to acquire biblical significance!

One nasty side effect of this ossification is that *yesterday's* best evidence drags down *today's* guidelines and clinical pathways. An example is the lowering of blood glucose in type 2 diabetes. For many years, the 'evidence-based' assumption was that the more intensively a person's blood glucose was controlled, the better the outcomes would be. But more recently, a large meta-analysis showed that intensive glucose control had no benefit over moderate control, but was associated with a twofold increase in the incidence of severe hypoglycaemia [13]. Yet, UK GPs were still being performance-managed through a scheme called the *Quality and Outcomes Framework* (QOF) to strive for intensive glucose control *after* the publication of that meta-analysis had shown an adverse benefit–harm ratio [14]. This is because it takes time for practice and policy to catch up with the evidence – but the existence of the QOF, introduced to make care more evidence-based, actually had the effect of making it *less* evidence-based!

Perhaps the most powerful criticism of EBM is that, if misapplied, it dismisses the patient's own perspective on the illness in favour of an average effect on a population sample or a column of quality-adjusted life-years (QALYs) (see Chapter 11) calculated by a medical statistician. Some writers on EBM are enthusiastic about using a decision-tree approach to incorporate the patient's perspective into an evidence-based treatment choice. In practice, this often proves impossible, because as I pointed out in Section 'The patient perspective', patients' experiences are complex stories that refuse to be reduced to a tree of yes/no (or 'therapy on, therapy off') decisions.

The (effective) imposition of standardised care reduces the clinician's ability to respond to the idiosyncratic, here-and-now issues emerging in a particular consultation. The very core of the EBM approach is to use a population average (or more accurately, an average from a representative sample) to inform decision-making for that patient. But as many others before me have pointed out, a patient is not a mean or a median but an individual, whose illness inevitably has unique and unclassifiable features. Not only does over-standardisation make the care offered less aligned to individual needs, it also de-skills the practitioner so that he or she loses the ability to customise and personalise care (or, in the case of recently trained clinicians, fails to gain that ability in the first place).

As Spence [1] put it, 'Evidence engenders a sense of absolutism, but absolutism is to be feared absolutely. "I can't go against the evidence" has produced our reductionist flowchart medicine, with thoughtless polypharmacy, especially in populations with comorbidity. Many thousands of people die directly from adverse drug reactions as a result'.

Let me give you another example. I recently undertook some research that required me to spend a long period of time watching junior doctors in an A&E Department. I discovered that whenever a child was seen with an injury, the junior doctor completed a set of questions on the electronic patient's record. These questions were based on an evidence-based guideline to rule out non-accidental injury. But because the young doctors filled these boxes for every child, it seemed to me that the 'hunch' that they might have had in the case of any *particular* child was absent. This standardised approach contrasted to my own junior doctor days 30 years ago, when we had no guidelines but spent quite a bit of our time playing and honing our hunches.

Another concern about 'EBM done well' is the sheer volume of evidence-based guidance and advice that now exists. As I pointed out in Section 'The great guidelines debate', the guidelines needed to manage the handful of patients seen on a typical 24-h acute take run to over 3000 pages and would require over a week of reading by a clinician [15]! And that does not include point-of-care prompting for other evidence-based interventions (e.g. risk factor management) in patients seen in a non-acute setting. For example, whenever I see a patient between 16 and 25 in general practice, a pop-up prompt tells me to 'offer chlamydia screening'. Some of my own qualitative work with Swinglehurst [16] has shown how disruptive such prompts are to the dynamic of the clinician–patient consultation.

A more philosophical criticism of EBM is that it is predicated on a simplistic and naïve version of what knowledge is. The assumption is that knowledge can be equated with 'facts' derived from research studies that can be formalised into guidelines and 'translated' (i.e. implemented by practitioners and policymakers). But as I have argued elsewhere, knowledge is a complex and uncertain beast [17]. For one thing, only some knowledge can be thought of as something an individual can know as a 'fact'; there is another level of knowledge that is *collective* – that is, socially shared and organisationally embedded [18]. As Tsoukas and Vladimirou [19] put it:

> *Knowledge is a flux mix of framed experiences, values, contextual information and expert insight that provides a framework for evaluating and incorporating new experiences and information. It originates and is applied in the minds of knowers. In organizations, it*

*often becomes embedded not only in documents or repositories but also
in organizational routines, processes, practices, and norms.*

Gabbay and May [20] illustrated this collective element of knowledge in
their study that I mentioned briefly in Section 'How can we help ensure
that evidence-based guidelines are followed?' on page 138. Whilst these
researchers, who watched GPs in action for several months, never observed
the doctors consulting guidelines directly, they did observe them discussing
and negotiating these guidelines among themselves and also acting in a
way that showed they had somehow absorbed and come to embody the
key components of many evidence-based guidelines 'by osmosis'. These
collectively embodied, socially shared elements of guidelines are what
Gabbay and May called *mindlines.*

Facts held by individuals (e.g. a research finding that one person has
discovered on a thorough literature search) may become collectivised
through a variety of mechanisms, including efforts to make it relevant to
colleagues (timely, salient, actionable), legitimate (credible, authoritative,
reasonable) and accessible (available, understandable, assimilable) and to
take account of the points of departure (assumptions, world views, priorities)
of a particular audience.

These mechanisms are elements of the science of knowledge translation – a
major topic that is beyond the scope of this book [17, 20–22]. The key point
here is that to present EBM purely as the sequence of individual tasks set
out in earlier chapters of this book is an over-simplistic depiction. If you are
comfortable with the basics of EBM, I strongly encourage you to go on to
pursue the literature on these wider dimensions of knowledge.

Why is 'evidence-based policymaking' so hard to achieve?

For some people, the main criticism of EBM is that it fails to get evidence simply and logically into policy. And the reason why policies don't flow simply
and logically from research evidence is that there are so many other factors involved.

Take the question of publicly funded treatments for infertility, for example.
You can produce a stack of evidence as high as a house to demonstrate
that intervention X leads to a take-home baby rate of Y% in women with
characteristics (such as age or comorbidity) Z, but that won't take the heat
out of the decision to sanction infertility treatment from a limited health
care budget. This was the question addressed by a Primary Care Trust
policymaking forum I attended recently, which had to balance this decision
against competing options (outreach support for first episode of psychosis

and a community-based diabetes specialist nurse for epilepsy). It wasn't that the members of the forum ignored the evidence – there was so much evidence in the background papers that the courier couldn't get it to fit through my letterbox – it was that values, rather than evidence, were what the final decision hung on. And as many have pointed out, policymaking is as much about the struggle to resolve conflicts of values in particular local or national contexts as it is about getting evidence into practice [23].

In other words, the policymaking process cannot be considered as a 'macro' version of the sequence depicted in Section 1.1 ('convert our information needs into answerable questions ... ' etc). Like other processes that fall under the heading 'politics' (with a small 'p'), policymaking is fundamentally about persuading one's fellow decision-makers of the superiority of one course of action over another. This model of the policymaking process is strongly supported by research studies, which suggest that at its heart lies unpredictability, ambiguity, and the possibility of alternative interpretations of the 'evidence' [23, 24].

The quest to make policymaking 'fully evidence based' may actually not be a desirable goal, as this benchmark arguably devalues democratic debate about the ethical and moral issues faced in policy choices. The 2005 UK Labour Party manifesto claimed that 'what matters is what works'. But what matters, surely, is not just what 'works', but what is appropriate in the circumstances, and what is agreed by society to be the overall desirable goal. Deborah Stone, in her book Policy Paradox, argues that much of the policy process involves debates about values masquerading as debates about facts and data. In her words: 'The essence of policymaking in political communities [is] the struggle over ideas. Ideas are at the centre of all political conflict ... Each idea is an argument, or more accurately, a collection of arguments in favour of different ways of seeing the world' [25].

One of the most useful theoretical papers on the use of evidence in health care policymaking is by Dobrow and colleagues [26]. They distinguish the philosophical-normative orientation (that there is an objective reality to be discovered and that a piece of 'evidence' can be deemed 'valid' and 'reliable' independent of the context in which it is to be used) from the practical-operational orientation, in which evidence is defined in relation to a specific decision-making context, is never static, and is characterised by emergence, ambiguity and incompleteness. From a practical-operational standpoint, research evidence is based on designs (such as randomised trials) that explicitly strip the study of contextual 'contaminants' and which therefore ignore the multiple, complex and interacting determinants of health. It follows that a complex intervention that 'works' in one setting at one time will not necessarily 'work' in a different setting at a different time, and one that proves 'cost-effective' in one setting will not necessarily provide value for money in a different setting. Many of the arguments raised about EBM in recent years have addressed precisely this controversy about the nature of knowledge.

Questioning the nature of evidence – and indeed, questioning evidential knowledge itself – is a somewhat scary place to end a basic introductory textbook on EBM, because most of the previous chapters in this book assume what Dobrow would call a philosophical-normative orientation. My own advice is this: if you are a humble student or clinician trying to pass your exams or do a better job at the bedside of individual patients, and if you feel thrown by the uncertainties I've raised in this final section, you can probably safely ignore them until you're actively involved in policymaking yourself. But if your career is at the stage when you're already sitting on decision-making bodies and trying to work out the answer to the question posed in the title to this section, I'd suggest you explore some of the papers and books referenced in this section. Do watch for the next generation of EBM research, which increasingly addresses the fuzzier and more contestible aspects of this important topic.

References

1 Spence D. Why evidence is bad for your health. BMJ: British Medical Journal 2010;**341**:c6368.
2 Timmermans S, Berg M. *The gold standard: the challenge of evidence-based medicine and standardization in health care.* Philadelphia: Temple University Press, 2003.
3 Timmermans S, Mauck A. The promises and pitfalls of evidence-based medicine. Health Affairs 2005;**24**(1):18–28.
4 Agoritsas T, Guyatt GH. Evidence-based medicine 20 years on: a view from the inside. The Canadian Journal of Neurological Sciences 2013;**40**(4):448–9.
5 Goldacre B. *Bad pharma: how drug companies mislead doctors and harm patients.* Random House Digital Inc., London, Fourth Estate, 2013.
6 Saukko PM, Farrimond H, Evans PH, et al. Beyond beliefs: risk assessment technologies shaping patients' experiences of heart disease prevention. Sociology of Health & Illness 2012;**34**(4):560–75.
7 Davis C, Abraham J. The socio-political roots of pharmaceutical uncertainty in the evaluation of 'innovative' diabetes drugs in the European Union and the US. Social Science & Medicine 2011;**72**(9):1574–81.
8 Jutel A. Framing disease: the example of female hypoactive sexual desire disorder. Social Science & Medicine 2010;**70**(7):1084–90.
9 Lugtenberg M, Burgers JS, Clancy C, et al. Current guidelines have limited applicability to patients with comorbid conditions: a systematic analysis of evidence-based guidelines. PloS One 2011;**6**(10):e25987.

10 Bull FC, Bauman AE. Physical inactivity: the "Cinderella" risk factor for non-communicable disease prevention. Journal of Health Communication 2011; 16(Suppl. 2):13–26.

11 Garcia-Moreno C, Watts C. Violence against women: an urgent public health priority. Bulletin of the World Health Organization 2011;89(1):2.

12 Clegg A, Young J, Iliffe S, et al. Frailty in elderly people. The Lancet 2013; 381:752–62.

13 Boussageon R, Bejan-Angoulvant T, Saadatian-Elahi M, et al. Effect of intensive glucose lowering treatment on all cause mortality, cardiovascular death, and microvascular events in type 2 diabetes: meta-analysis of randomised controlled trials. BMJ: British Medical Journal 2011;343:d4169.

14 Calvert M, Shankar A, McManus RJ, et al. Effect of the quality and outcomes framework on diabetes care in the United Kingdom: retrospective cohort study. BMJ: British Medical Journal 2009;338:b1870.

15 Allen D, Harkins K. Too much guidance? The Lancet 2005;365(9473):1768.

16 Swinglehurst D, Roberts C, Greenhalgh T. Opening up the 'black box' of the electronic patient record: a linguistic ethnographic study in general practice. Communication & Medicine 2011;8(1):3–15.

17 Greenhalgh T. What is this knowledge that we seek to "exchange"? The Milbank Quarterly 2010;88(4):492–9 doi: 10.1111/j.1468-0009.2010.00610.x[published Online First: Epub Date].

18 Contandriopoulos D, Lemire M, DENIS JL, et al. Knowledge exchange processes in organizations and policy arenas: a narrative systematic review of the literature. Milbank Quarterly 2010;88(4):444–83.

19 Tsoukas H, Vladimirou E. What is organizational knowledge? Journal of Management Studies 2001;38(7):973–3.

20 Gabbay J, May Al. Evidence based guidelines or collectively constructed "mindlines?" Ethnographic study of knowledge management in primary care. BMJ: British Medical Journal 2004;329(7473):1013.

21 Greenhalgh T, Wieringa S. Is it time to drop the 'knowledge translation' metaphor? A critical literature review. Journal of the Royal Society of Medicine 2011; 104(12):501–9 doi: 10.1258/jrsm.2011.110285[published Online First: Epub Date].

22 Graham ID, Logan J, Harrison MB, et al. Lost in knowledge translation: time for a map? Journal of Continuing Education in the Health Professions 2006; 26(1):13–24.

23 Greenhalgh T, Russell J. Evidence-based policymaking: a critique. Perspectives in Biology and Medicine 2009;52(2):304–18.

24 Scheel I, Hagen K, Oxman A. The unbearable lightness of healthcare policy making: a description of a process aimed at giving it some weight. Journal of Epidemiology and Community Health 2003;57(7):483–7.

25 Stone DA. Policy paradox: the art of political decision making. New York: WW Norton, 1997.

26 Dobrow MJ, Goel V, Upshur R. Evidence-based health policy: context and utilisation. Social Science & Medicine 2004;58(1):207–17.

Appendix 1 Checklists for finding, appraising and implementing evidence

Unless otherwise stated, these checklists can be applied to randomised controlled trials, other controlled clinical trials, cohort studies, case–control studies, or any other research evidence.

Is my practice evidence-based? – a context-sensitive checklist for individual clinical encounters (see Chapter 1)

1. Have I identified and prioritised the clinical, psychological, social, and other problem(s), taking into account the patient's perspective?
2. Have I performed a sufficiently competent and complete examination to establish the likelihood of competing diagnoses?
3. Have I considered additional problems and risk factors that may need opportunistic attention?
4. Have I, where necessary, sought evidence (from systematic reviews, guidelines, clinical trials and other sources) pertaining to the problems?
5. Have I assessed and taken into account the completeness, quality and strength of the evidence?
6. Have I applied valid and relevant evidence to this particular set of problems in a way that is both scientifically justified and intuitively sensible?
7. Have I presented the pros and cons of different options to the patient in a way they can understand, and incorporated the patient's preferences into the final recommendation?
8. Have I arranged review, recall, referral or other further care as necessary?

Checklist for searching (see Chapter 2)

1. Decide on the purpose of your search: browsing, seeking an answer to a clinical question, or a comprehensive review (e.g. prior to undertaking a piece of research), and design your search strategy accordingly (Section 'What are you looking for?').

2. Go for the highest level of evidence you can (Section 'Levels upon levels of evidence'). For example, high-quality synthesised sources (e.g. systematic reviews and evidence-based summaries and syntheses such as Clinical Evidence or NICE guidelines, Section 'Synthesised sources: systems, summaries and syntheses') represent a very high level of evidence.

3. For keeping abreast of new developments, use synopses such as POEMS ('patient-oriented evidence that matters'), *ACP Journal Club* or *Evidence-Based Medicine* journal (Section 'Pre-appraised sources: synopses of systematic reviews and primary studies').

4. Make yourself familiar with the specialised resources in your own field and use these routinely (Section 'Specialised resources').

5. When searching the Medline database for primary research, you will greatly increase the efficiency of your search if you do two broad searches and then combine them, or if you use tools such as the 'limit set' or 'clinical queries' function (Section 'Primary studies – tackling the jungle').

6. A very powerful way of identifying recent publications on a topic is to 'citation chain' an older paper (i.e. use a special electronic database to find which later papers have cited the older paper, Section 'Primary studies – tackling the jungle').

7. Federated search engines such as TRIP or SUMsearch search multiple resources simultaneously and are free (Section 'One-stop shopping: federated search engines').

8. Human sources (expert librarians, experts in the field) are an important component of a thorough search (Section 'Asking for help and asking around').

9. To improve your skill and confidence in searching, try an online self-study course (Section 'Online tutorials for effective searching').

Checklist to determine what a paper is about (see Chapter 3)

1. Why was the study performed (what clinical question did it address)?

2. What type of study was performed?
   - Primary research (experiment, randomised controlled trial, other controlled clinical trial, cohort study, case–control study, cross-sectional survey, longitudinal survey, case report, or case series)?

- Secondary research (simple overview, systematic review, meta-analysis, decision analysis, guideline development, economic analysis)?
3. Was the study design appropriate to the broad field of research addressed (therapy, diagnosis, screening, prognosis, causation)?
4. Did the study meet expected standards of ethics and governance?

Checklist for the methods section of a paper (see Chapter 4)

1. Was the study original?
2. Whom is the study about?
   - How were participants recruited?
   - Who was included in, and who was excluded from, the study?
   - Were the participants studied in 'real-life' circumstances?
3. Was the design of the study sensible?
   - What intervention or other manoeuvre was being considered?
   - What outcome(s) were measured, and how?
4. Was the study adequately controlled?
   - If a 'randomised trial', was randomisation truly random?
   - If a cohort, case–control or other non-randomised comparative study, were the controls appropriate?
   - Were the groups comparable in all important aspects except for the variable being studied?
   - Was assessment of outcome (or, in a case–control study, allocation of caseness) 'blind'?
5. Was the study large enough, and continued for long enough, and was follow-up complete enough, to make the results credible?

Checklist for the statistical aspects of a paper (see Chapter 5)

1. Have the authors set the scene correctly?
   - Have they determined whether their groups are comparable, and, if necessary, adjusted for baseline differences?
   - What sort of data have they got, and have they used appropriate statistical tests?
   - If the statistical tests in the paper are obscure, why have the authors chosen to use them?
   - Have the data been analysed according to the original study protocol?
2. Paired data, tails and outliers
   - Were paired tests performed on paired data?

- Was a two-tailed test performed whenever the effect of an intervention could conceivably be a negative one?
- Were outliers analysed with both common sense and appropriate statistical adjustments?
3. Correlation, regression and causation
   - Has correlation been distinguished from regression, and has the correlation coefficient ('r-value') been calculated and interpreted correctly?
   - Have assumptions been made about the nature and direction of causality?
4. Probability and confidence
   - Have 'p-values' been calculated and interpreted appropriately?
   - Have confidence intervals been calculated and do the authors' conclusions reflect them?
5. Have the authors expressed their results in terms of the likely harm or benefit that an individual patient can expect, such as
   - relative risk reduction;
   - absolute risk reduction;
   - number needed to treat?

Checklist for material provided by a pharmaceutical company representative (see Chapter 6)

See particularly Table 6.1 for questions on randomised trials based on the CONSORT statement

1. Does this material cover a subject that is clinically important in my practice?
2. Has this material been published in independent peer-reviewed journals? Has any significant evidence been omitted from this presentation or withheld from publication?
3. Does the material include high-level evidence such as systematic reviews, meta-analyses, or double-blind randomised controlled trials against the drug's closest competitor given at optimal dosage?
4. Have the trials or reviews addressed a clearly focused, important and answerable clinical question that reflects a problem of relevance to patients? Do they provide evidence on safety, tolerability, efficacy and price?
5. Has each trial or meta-analysis defined the condition to be treated, the patients to be included, the interventions to be compared and the outcomes to be examined?
6. Does the material provide direct evidence that the drug will help my patients live a longer, healthier, more productive and symptom-free life?

7. If a surrogate outcome measure has been used, what is the evidence that it is reliable, reproducible, sensitive, specific, a true predictor of disease and rapidly reflects the response to therapy?
8. Do trial results indicate whether (and how) the effectiveness of the treatments differed and whether there was a difference in the type or frequency of adverse reactions? Are the results expressed in terms of numbers needed to treat, and are they clinically as well as statistically significant?
9. If large amounts of material have been provided by the representative, which three papers provide the strongest evidence for the company's claims?

Checklist for a paper describing a study of a complex intervention (see Chapter 7)

1. What is the problem for which this complex intervention is seen as a possible solution?
2. What was done in the developmental phase of the research to inform the design of the complex intervention?
3. What were the core and non-core components of the intervention?
4. What was the theoretical mechanism of action of the intervention?
5. What outcome measures were used, and were these sensible?
6. What were the findings?
7. What process evaluation was performed – and what were the key findings of this?
8. If the findings were negative, to what extent can this be explained by implementation failure and/or inadequate optimisation of the intervention?
9. If the findings varied across different subgroups, to what extent have the authors explained this by refining their theory of change?
10. What further research do the authors believe is needed, and is this justified?

Checklist for a paper that claims to validate a diagnostic or screening test (see Chapter 8)

1. Is this test potentially relevant to my practice?
2. Has the test been compared with a true gold standard?
3. Did this validation study include an appropriate spectrum of participants?
4. Has work-up bias been avoided?
5. Has observer bias been avoided?

6. Was the test shown to be reproducible both within and between observers?
7. What are the features of the test as derived from this validation study?
8. Were confidence intervals given for sensitivity, specificity and other features of the test?
9. Has a sensible 'normal range' been derived from these results?
10. Has this test been placed in the context of other potential tests in the diagnostic sequence for the condition?

Checklist for a systematic review or meta-analysis (see Chapter 9)

1. Did the review address an important clinical question?
2. Was a thorough search carried out of the appropriate database(s) and were other potentially important sources explored?
3. Was methodological quality (especially factors that might predispose to bias) assessed and the trials weighted accordingly?
4. How sensitive are the results to the way the review has been performed?
5. Have the numerical results been interpreted with common sense and due regard to the broader aspects of the problem?

Checklist for a set of clinical guidelines (see Chapter 10)

1. Did the preparation and publication of these guidelines involve a significant conflict of interest?
2. Are the guidelines concerned with an appropriate topic, and do they state clearly the goal of ideal treatment in terms of health and/or cost outcome?
3. Was a specialist in the methodology of secondary research (e.g. meta-analyst) involved?
4. Have all the relevant data been scrutinised and are guidelines' conclusions in keeping with the data?
5. Do they address variations in clinical practice and other controversial areas (e.g. optimum care in response to genuine or perceived underfunding)?
6. Are the guidelines valid and reliable?
7. Are they clinically relevant, comprehensive, and flexible?
8. Do they take into account what is acceptable to, affordable by, and practically possible for patients?
9. Do they include recommendations for their own dissemination, implementation and periodic review?

Checklist for an economic analysis (see Chapter 11)

1. Is the analysis based on a study that answers a clearly-defined clinical question about an economically important issue?
2. Whose viewpoint are costs and benefits being considered from?
3. Have the interventions being compared been shown to be clinically effective?
4. Are the interventions sensible and workable in the settings where they are likely to be applied?
5. Which method of economic analysis was used, and was this appropriate?
   - if the interventions produced identical outcomes ⇒ cost-minimisation analysis;
   - if the important outcome is unidimensional ⇒ cost-effectiveness analysis;
   - if the important outcome is multidimensional ⇒ cost-utility analysis;
   - if the cost–benefit equation for this condition needs to be compared with cost–benefit equations for different conditions ⇒ cost-benefit analysis;
   - if a cost–benefit analysis would otherwise be appropriate but the preference values given to different health states are disputed or likely to change ⇒ cost-consequences analysis.
6. How were costs and benefits measured?
7. Were incremental, rather than absolute, benefits compared?
8. Was health status in the 'here and now' given precedence over health status in the distant future?
9. Was a sensitivity analysis performed?
10. Were 'bottom-line' aggregate scores overused?

Checklist for a qualitative research paper (see Chapter 12)

1. Did the article describe an important clinical problem addressed via a clearly formulated question?
2. Was a qualitative approach appropriate?
3. How were (i) the setting and (ii) the participants selected?
4. What was the researcher's perspective, and has this been taken into account?
5. What methods did the researcher use for collecting data – and are these described in enough detail?
6. What methods did the researcher use to analyse the data – and what quality control measures were implemented?

7. Are the results credible, and if so, are they clinically important?
8. What conclusions were drawn, and are they justified by the results?
9. Are the findings of the study transferable to other clinical settings?

Checklist for a paper describing questionnaire research (see Chapter 13)

1. What did the researchers want to find out, and was a questionnaire the most appropriate research design?
2. If an 'off the peg' questionnaire (i.e. a previously published and validated one) was available, did the researchers use it (and if not, why not)?
3. What claims have the researchers made about the validity of the questionnaire (its ability to measure what they want it to measure) and reliability (its ability to give consistent results across time and within/between researchers)? Are these claims justified?
4. Was the questionnaire appropriately structured and presented, and were the items worded appropriately for the sensitivity of the subject area and the health literacy of the respondents?
5. Were adequate instructions and explanations included?
6. Was the questionnaire adequately piloted, and was the definitive version amended in the light of pilot results?
7. Was the sample of potential participants appropriately selected, large enough and representative enough?
8. How was the questionnaire distributed (e.g. by post, email, telephone) and administered (self completion, researcher-assisted completion), and were these approaches appropriate?
9. Were the needs of particular subgroups taken into account in the design and administration of the questionnaire? For example, what was done to capture the perspective of illiterate respondents or those speaking a different language from the researcher?
10. What was the response rate, and why? If the response rate was low (<70%), have the researchers shown that no systematic differences existed between responders and non-responders?
11. What sort of analysis was carried out on the questionnaire data, and was this appropriate? Is there any evidence of 'data dredging' – that is, analyses that were not hypothesis driven?
12. What were the results? Were they definitive (statistically significant), and were important negative and non-significant results also reported?
13. Have qualitative data (e.g. free text responses) been adequately interpreted (e.g. using an explicit theoretical framework). Have quotes been

used judiciously to illustrate more general findings rather than to add drama?

14. What do the results mean and have the researchers drawn an appropriate link between the data and their conclusions?

Checklist for a paper describing a quality improvement study (see Chapter 14)

1. What was the context?
2. What was the aim of the study?
3. What was the mechanism by which the authors hoped to improve quality?
4. Was the intended quality improvement initiative evidence-based?
5. How did the authors measure success, and was this reasonable?
6. How much detail was given on the change process, and what insights can be gleaned from this?
7. What were the main findings?
8. What was the explanation for the success, failure or mixed fortunes of the initiative – and was this reasonable?
9. In the light of the findings, what do the authors feel are the next steps in the quality improvement cycle locally?
10. What did the authors claim to be the generalisable lessons for other teams, and was this reasonable?

Checklist for health care organisations working towards an evidence-based culture for clinical and purchasing decisions (see Chapter 15)

1. *Leadership*: How often has effectiveness information or evidence-based medicine been discussed at board meetings in the last 12 months? Has the board taken time out to learn about developments in clinical and cost-effectiveness?
2. *Investment*: What resources is the organisation investing in finding and using clinical effectiveness information? Is there a planned approach to promoting evidence-based medicine that is properly resourced and staffed?
3. *Policies and guidelines*: Who is responsible for receiving, acting on and monitoring the implementation of evidence-based guidance and policy recommendations such as NICE guidance or Effective Health Care Bulletins? What action has been taken on each of these publications issued

to date? Do arrangements ensure that both managers and clinicians play their part in guideline development and implementation?

4. *Training*: Has any training been provided to staff within the organisation (both clinical and non-clinical) on appraising and using evidence of effectiveness to influence clinical practice?

5. *Contracts*: How often does clinical and cost-effectiveness information form an important part of contract negotiation and agreement? How many contracts contain terms that set out how effectiveness information is to be used?

6. *Incentives*: What incentives – both individual and organisational – exist to encourage the practice of evidence-based medicine? What disincentives exist to discourage inappropriate practice and unjustified variations in clinical decision-making?

7. *Information systems*: Is the potential of existing information systems to monitor clinical effectiveness being used to the full? Is there a business case for new information systems to address the task, and is this issue being considered when IT purchasing decisions are made?

8. *Clinical audit*: Is there an effective clinical audit programme throughout the organisation, capable of addressing issues of clinical effectiveness and bringing about appropriate changes in practice?

Appendix 2 **Assessing the effects of an intervention**

	Outcome event		Total
	Yes	No	
Control group	a	b	a+b
Experimental group	c	d	c+d

If outcome event is undesirable (e.g. death)
CER = risk of undesirable outcome in control group = $a/(a + b)$
EER = risk of undesirable outcome in experimental group = $c/(c + d)$
Relative risk of undesirable event in experimental versus control group = EER/CER
Absolute risk reduction in treated group (ARR) = CER − EER
Number needed to treat (NNT) = 1/ARR = 1/(CER − EER)

If outcome event is desirable (e.g. cure)
CER = risk of desirable outcome in control group = $a/(a + b)$
EER = risk of desirable outcome in experimental group = $c/(c + d)$
Relative benefit increase in treated versus control group = EER/CER
Absolute benefit increase in treated versus control group = EER − CER
Number needed to treat (NNT) = 1/ARR = 1/(EER − CER)

Acknowledgement

Thanks to Paul Glasziou from the Oxford Centre for Evidence-Based Medicine for clarification on these concepts.

How to Read a Paper: The Basics of Evidence-Based Medicine, Fifth Edition. Trisha Greenhalgh.
© 2014 John Wiley & Sons, Ltd. Published 2014 by John Wiley & Sons, Ltd.

Index